Clinical cases in dietetics

Clinical cases in dietetics

Dr Fred Pender

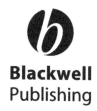

Blackwell
Publishing

Blackwell Publishing editorial offces:
Blackwell Publishing Ltd, 9600 Garsington Road, Oxford OX4 2DQ, UK
Tel: +44 (0)1865 776868
Blackwell Publishing Professional, 2121 State Avenue, Ames, Iowa 50014-8300, USA
Tel: +1 515 292 0140
Blackwell Publishing Asia Pty Ltd, 550 Swanston Street, Carlton, Victoria 3053, Australia
Tel: +61 (0)3 8359 1011

First published 2008 by Blackwell Publishing Ltd
2 2010
ISBN: 9781405125642

Library of Congress Cataloging-in-Publication Data
Pender, F. (Frederic)
Clinical cases in dietetics / Fred Pender.
p. ; cm
Includes bibliographical references and index.
ISBN-13: 978-1-4051-2564-2 (pbk. : alk. paper)
ISBN-10: 1-4051-2564-0 (pbk. : alk. paper)   1. Dietetics–Case studies.
2. Dietetics–Problems, exercises, etc.   I. Title.
[DNLM: 1. Diet Therapy–methods–Case Reports.   2. Diet Therapy–methods–Problems and Exercises.   3. Dietetics–methods–Case Reports.   4. Dietetics–methods–Problems and Exercises.   WB 18.2 P397c 2008]

RM216.P412 2008
613.2–dc22

2007036833

A catalogue record for this title is available from the British Library

Set in 10 on 12 pt Avenir
by SNP Best-set Typesetter Ltd., Hong Kong

FSC
Mixed Sources
Product group from well-managed
forests and other controlled sources
Cert no. SGS-COC-2953
www.fsc.org
© 1996 Forest Stewardship Council

For further information on Blackwell Publishing, visit our website:
www.blackwellpublishing.com

Contents

The diaries (and contexts) 103

The referrals (and contexts) 119

The mini-cases (and contexts)   135

The commentaries   141

The appendices: clinical information and reference data   231

The appendices: tools   **265**

The introduction

A casebook approach

The practice of dietetics is primarily concerned with the practitioner who is presented with personal, medical, biochemical, physical and other data or information from patients or clients, and who subsequently arrives at a reasoned clinical judgement based on this information. This judgement can then be used as a basis for dietary intervention. The diverse nature of the client group, together with the range of presenting signs and symptoms and other clinical information pose for the student practitioner the challenges of using these data to inform the clinical decision-making process.

This textbook takes the reader through the process of therapeutic thinking, to result in considered solutions about practical clinical dietary intervention. The approach involves development of critical thinking and the skills of clinical detection. The reader is presented with a series of clinical cases of varying complexity and range. The text encourages the reader to consider each patient as a unique collection of data to be worked through. Each case includes a commentary (towards the end of the book), opportunities for reflection on practice and key learning points.

Preface

As the need for healthcare practitioners to demonstrate competence and meet standards of proficiency increases, making professional judgements based on clinical reasoning becomes crucial. The process of clinical reasoning begins with the working through of clinical, social and other information so that judgements can be made in a systematic, logical and consistent manner to arrive at an informed position that can be used as the basis for therapeutic care or intervention strategy. Thus, delivery of advice to a patient or client is rooted in a process of investigational skills that considers fully the context in which the client is placed as opposed to a more traditional approach – basing interventional practice merely on the knowledge of the patient or client's medical condition.

The formulation of dietary advice is therefore based on the outcome of examination of data presented by the client, which are elicited using a systematic approach. This considered approach has many advantages: it allows full exploration of the client's context and thus dietary advice can be individually tailored; it avoids the pitfall of delivering advice in a habitual, ritualistic and less meaningful way; it encourages development of systematic investigational technique by the student practitioner and promotes engagement with the subject, client and client contexts. Ultimately it will result in instinctive professional behaviour that is evidence based and applies to the client in question.

The investigational approach in a student dietitian begins at an early stage in their learning career, where the student is first exposed to data and their management. As the student begins to apply knowledge and engage with clinical information, there is clearly a need to develop skills to manage these processes. In programmes of study involving placement of a student in a clinical learning environment, these processes need to begin early and be developed over time. Ideally, to effect good intervention practice, the student dietitian needs to have these *clinical skills* firmly in place before clinical exposure. It is the contention of the author that the process of effective critical and clinical thinking, reasoning and decision-making begins early in the pre-registration programme, before practice placement, and that the process is assisted with the use of case studies that focus on problems or issues.

It is the intention of this series of cases to assist the student of dietetics to engage more instinctively with clinical information. Dietetics is not an exact science; it has to deal with the vagaries of the human subject and the social and disease contexts, and draws on investigational attributes of the practitioner to effect good professional practice. The basis of this textbook rests on presenting the student with information, encouraging an investigational approach in managing the information and developing interpretational skills to arrive at a reasoned, professional judgement.

Experience suggests that students of dietetics need to place dietetics in the holistic context of the practice field, bringing in ethical, political, social and clinical dimensions; rote learning is neither useful nor wise and students of dietetics need to demonstrate problem solving as one of their *clinical skills* prior to placement and in practice. It serves to encourage instinctive and evidence-based practice; if the process is cultured in a student practitioner, even if the knowledge base changes, the process encourages the student to deliver health care based on evidence and unique data presented by the client. Further, it assists the student in planning and prioritising care for a client.

The cases presented in this textbook are predominantly taken from clinical experience and have been altered only to protect the confidentiality of the client or referral agent. The cases are therefore largely real, and represent accurately the scope and variety of questions posed in clinical practice. Each case has been subsequently worked through by both specialist practitioners and students; the resultant cases are therefore *tried and tested examples* of the problems presented to the dietitian in clinical or primary care practice.

Introduction

The cases presented in this textbook represent the scope and level of problems met in community and clinical practice of the dietitian. The cases challenge the student with 'virtual' or simulated situations intended to closely match issues that occur in routine professional practice. In the learning centre or university, student practitioners are guided by academic theory essentially involving class work where there is a greater or lesser degree of student independence.

Theoretical grounding is the basis of learning as a prelude to clinical life; case study work supports formal instruction by providing illustrations to which theory can be applied. Indeed, some medical schools now use case study illustration as the core method of instruction – theoretical underpinning guided by acquisition of knowledge on a *needs to know* basis as the medical student engages with cases. Understanding, as opposed to knowledge acquisition, is more easily demonstrated in applied learning situations, an example of which is the case study. It encourages the process of critical thinking and clinical reasoning and therefore fosters the problem-solving approach. The approach taken in this textbook is to encourage the student *how to think* (a skill) and not *what to think* (a knowledge base); these concepts stimulate the process of systematic enquiry resulting in better-informed clinical judgements.

The intention is that students need to *use* this book. Case studies, by their very nature, are activities and involve the student in processing information in a logical sequence of steps. Case studies need to be used alongside theory which may be delivered formally as part of a lecture programme or the cases themselves can stimulate the learner to seek the theoretical underpinning.

Active learning is about engaging the student in issues and fostering a questioning attitude. This textbook assists, therefore, in the development of a clinical detective.

How to use this book

The cases are presented in many ways and different formats, but essentially there is a piece of prose (the stem of the case) that takes the form of a whole case, a letter of referral or the patient history. The stem or 'story' sets the scene and begins to unfold issues that the student has to deal with, such as the client's social and socio-economic background and significant history (clinical and physical information). Following the 'story' or scenario, the student is guided by a series of questions to extract relevant pieces of the story that may be significant in generating solutions or solving issues.

The book has several uses: it may be used for self-study when the student wishes to work through the cases unassisted; it may assist the student's formal learning if the tutor uses the cases to extend theoretical aspects of learning into practical areas. It may be used as the stimulus for learning and form the spine of a practical course in which theory may be guided by the problems. In addition, the cases can be used by individual students or as part of group working, where small syndicates of students may work through the problems. Some cases may be suitable for assessing students formatively or summatively; some may be useful for formal course-work assignments.

Whilst one of the intentions is to use this textbook as a self-study framework, it is always useful to come together with either the tutor or peers to discuss findings. Others' interpretations of problems are always useful in clarifying or fine-tuning the detail of the case or the outcomes generated. In addition, this encourages a student to engage in critical debate and foster group-working skills.

Each case or problem is accompanied by an explanatory commentary (potential answers) that attempts to provide a framework or learning skeleton for the 'answers' or solutions (see below for a fuller explanation). The discussions in the commentaries are by no means exhaustive and other important issues or questions may be examined; some issues and perspectives may not be mentioned or examined in any depth.

Making the most of the cases

Each case presents the student with information that may or may not pose issues or problems. This stimulates the student to move from baseline information through a series of logical steps to arrive at a judgement (solution or answer). Arriving at a clinical judgement involves using a combination of clinical and social information and placing this into the therapeutic context of the client or patient by relating this to evidence-based published clinical guidelines. This sequence of events utilises the process of clinical reasoning (Figure 1).

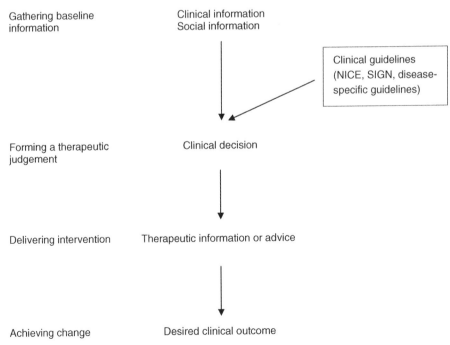

Gathering baseline information	Clinical information Social information
	Clinical guidelines (NICE, SIGN, disease-specific guidelines)
Forming a therapeutic judgement	Clinical decision
Delivering intervention	Therapeutic information or advice
Achieving change	Desired clinical outcome

Figure 1 Process of clinical reasoning. NICE, National Institute for Health and Clinical Excellence; SIGN, Scottish Intercollegiate Guidelines Network.

As a result of this process, therapeutic information can be informed and relevant. Appropriate dietary advice can be formulated and ultimately delivered to the client or patient, using an evidence-based, clinical guideline framework. At the end of the stage or episode of care, the desired or preferred clinical outcome may be achieved.

What you will need

To maximise the learning experience presented in the cases, it is important to become familiar with the predictable variables of each case: the medical condition, the evidence-based therapeutic and dietetic care, the pharmacological management of the condition and the agreed best practice or evidence-based practice for dietary or nutritional intervention (published disease-specific clinical guidelines). Thus, to assist your learning, you should have access to:

- A substantial dietetic text (*Manual of Dietetic Practice*, 4th edn. 2007).
- A substantial medical text (e.g. *Davidson's Principles and Practice of Medicine* (Churchill Livingstone); *Kumar and Clark's Clinical Medicine* (Elsevier Saunders)).
- A substantial text of drugs: use and metabolism, such as the *British National Formulary* (*BNF*) or *Monthly Index of Medical Specialities* (*MIMS*).
- Published clinical guidelines (hard copy) or those available on the Internet (be sure to use a peer-reviewed or scientifically regulated website).

Prior to starting each case the student may wish to familiarise him- or herself with their university notes, specific chapters of the *Manual* and the clinical biochemistry/ physiology/ pathology/ pharmacology texts that underpin the cases.

For full forms of abbreviations used in the text please see Appendix 7.

Making sense of the clinical information

Essentially, arriving at a clinical judgement involves interpreting data or working through clinical information. This information comes from several sources: the patient, in the course of a therapeutic interview; the physician or medical team member, and from documentation written about the patient in case notes (or notes). Documentation in notes may be descriptive and inform about the history of the patient or may accurately report the results of clinical tests (numerical blood and urine values, and other requested information).

Information presented in this casebook includes both descriptive and accurate clinical information about each case. The descriptive information attempts to capture the history and context of the patient or client; the clinical data reflect the results of tests requested on behalf of the patient to assist with making a therapeutic judgement. Descriptive or qualitative information helps to guide a practitioner towards a judgement; the accurate or more quantitative information or clinical data assist in confirming a judgement or focusing on issues to resolve. Each case requires the reader to make sense of the clinical information, in the context described. Some information included is recorded in imperial measures; other data are given as metric values. This has been deliberately done to reflect the range of recorded measurements encountered in practice.

Interpretation of the clinical chemistry

Clinical information is used by the medical or surgical team to:

- confirm a diagnosis;
- assist in determining differential diagnosis (distinguishing between a number of potential diagnoses);
- refine a diagnosis;
- assess the stage or progress of the disease or condition;
- monitor the presence of side-effects or the effectiveness of therapeutic intervention.

In the hospital or primary care setting, clinical chemistry laboratories analyse samples of human products (for example, blood or urine), for the various analytes of interest, usually at the request of the physician, surgeon or a member of the therapeutic team. Data or clinical information is recorded on reports issued by the laboratory and included for reference in the patient's notes; members of the therapeutic team use selected clinical information to inform the therapeutic management of the patient or client.

Clinical information is usually expressed as a numerical value of the concentration or activity in appropriate units. The values may then be used to assess the patient or client's status, by comparing them with reference standards. Laboratories present information against these standards, in a standardised format. Student practitioners need to become familiar with usual reference standards (see Appendix 6) and the potential meaning of values that fall below, within or above reference standards. Understanding the extent to which the clinical results move away from the reference standard range and the clinical importance of this requires experience and careful interpretation. The student needs to study the clinical biochemistry and the disease-specific pathological factors which may affect concentrations of serum/plasma parameters.

It must be remembered that whilst analytical determination of the various blood parameters is highly accurate, the techniques may be hampered by other factors and some results may be rendered inaccurate with reporting of spurious values. The student practitioner must recognise the sources of variation in results, and these can be found in textbooks of clinical biochemistry. The major sources of variation are analytical error, mislabelled serial results of the same patient, biological causes and within- and between-person variation.

Clinical data must be interpreted in the context of the patient's history and presenting features. Subjective information may be useful in putting the patient or client's clinical information in context. It is usual, however, to relate the patient or client's results to 'reference standards'. These standards have been derived from a reference population and usually in the context of healthy individuals. Reference standards may also be derived from a defined population of disease-specific individuals although most commonly reference standards of ranges obtained from a healthy population are used, and this is generally assumed. To interpret results accurately, knowledge of the following is important:

- the reference range for healthy individuals, relative to appropriate age and sex;
- the reference range of values to be expected in the reference-disease population;
- the prevalence of the disease in the population to which the patient or client belongs;
- the level of hydration of the client, especially where hydration status may fluctuate (as is the case with the older person).

Getting started

It is important to fully understand the concepts involved in the process of clinical reasoning. The analytical process requires the student to engage with information at various stages. The cases in this book will essentially guide the student through this process.

Each case presents the student with a patient or client history, which includes a scenario or stem of medical, physical and social information that sets the client in context. The stem includes some recent history and represents information that is current or fresh, which helps to inform the student practitioner of contemporary issues facing the client. The study questions (Questions to consider) guide the student through a profitable route to engage with the process of clinical reasoning and thus attempt to resolve issues presented in the case. Study questions assist in general exploration of some key concepts related to each case. These questions may be tackled before solving the case, forming a useful theoretical basis to help formulate potential solutions to problems.

Cases presented in the referral or diary sections should be dealt with similarly, except that the information is set out slightly differently. Solutions to individual cases are not exhaustive and the commentaries provide a guide to best practice suggestions. The commentaries are taken from views of dietitians and students presented with the cases during the piloting of this textbook. They attempt to capture the principal ingredients of potential solutions to cases.

Adopting an analytical approach to the cases

Use of a logical, stepwise approach to solving cases encourages the student to be consistent when making judgements. The following 'model' uses an efficient, practical approach to case work, and takes the student through the significant processes in problem solving.

Step	Stages and commentary
1	**Stem (case or problem)** Read the case through and check and clarify any unfamiliar terminology or information
2	**Key information** Identify significant data or information provided in the stem
3	**Brainstorm** Explore the case and identify key issues thought to contribute to solving the case
4	**Resources** Identify key sources of information useful in addressing the case (current clinical guidelines, reference data)
5	**Plan** Make a preliminary judgement about the case and devise a therapeutic plan
6	**Defend the judgement** Confirm the initial judgement using appropriate evidence and reference criteria
7	**Communicate the judgement** Decide on the most appropriate method to record the solution (for example, care plan, prescribed notation unless otherwise directed)
8	**Reflection** Consider the process and how near you got to most points given in the commentary on the case. What issues did it raise? Put together an action plan to improve your problem-solving or case-related skills

Adopting an analytical approach to the diaries

Some things are important to remember when examining the diet diaries (including symptom or activity record). First, they are useful self-monitoring tools. Clients record and begin to engage with specific intake of food and drink and dietary behaviour associated with the intake, and therefore they may begin to understand the importance of the dietary intake or behaviour associated with their condition. Second, diaries are usually completed by interested individuals and are usually not as subject to bias as other methods of assessment of dietary intake. Thus, records may give a truer picture of actual or habitual intakes and behaviour.

Approaches to scrutinising diaries may include:

- a quantitative scan (comparing *actual* portion or serving sizes with *average* portion or serving sizes) – making a judgement about eating regularity and eating behaviours;
- a qualitative scan (comparing intakes of servings from food groups against those recommended nationally in a healthy eating model intake, such as the Balance of Good Health);
- investigating any possible relationship between symptoms, behaviour or clinical signs with key nutrients, foods or aspects of dietary intake (including behaviour);
- assessing lifestyle characteristics against government targets (physical activity and intake of alcohol);
- formulating dietary, nutritional or lifestyle approaches for the client to assist with clinical control or improvement in quality of life (reduction in symptoms);
- offering advice to meet nutritional or lifestyle goals.

It should be remembered that dietary records may not always be completed adequately (for example omission of portion sizes and some qualitative information) but diary entries can be clarified with the client at the first therapeutic interview. With this method of dietary assessment, making assumptions is inevitable (for example, does the intake reflect habitual intake?), but this can also be clarified with the client.

Adopting an analytical approach to the referrals

Referrals for dietary advice or a dietary consultation are usually brief and may take the form of a letter, a specific request form or nutritional screening tool. A helpful approach here may be to highlight the facts you are told (underscore or note) and begin to think about key issues presented by the case. Since the referral is usually a prelude to a first consultation with the patient or client to initiate or continue care, it is useful to piece together the known information and think about what additional information would help inform the approach to be taken with the client. It is also helpful to prioritise the key issues to be discussed or explored so that the consultation can be anticipated and planned strategically.

Acknowledgements

This textbook is a collection of real-life clinical stories taken from practice. Names of clients and patients referred to have been replaced with fictitious names to protect their identity. Special thanks are extended to those who have given so generously of their experiences. Grateful thanks are also given to those practitioners who have helped with formulating possible solutions (commentaries) to the cases. They include:

Nadia Aslam, Nutrition Support Dietitian
Royal Blackburn Hospital, Blackburn

Elizabeth Bridcut, Advanced Dietitian
Wirral Hospital NHS Trust, Arrowe Park Hospital

Victoria Driver, Specialist Dietitian
East Lancashire Primary Care Trust

Kirstine Farrer, Consultant Dietitian (Intestinal Failure)
Salford PCT and Salford Royal NHS Trust, Manchester

Laura Forrest, Diabetes Community Dietitian
Pennine Acute NHS Trust

Paul Greene, Cardiac Dietitian
North East Wales NHS Trust, Wrexham

Amanda Hamilton, Specialist Dietitian
Macclesfield District General Hospital

Elizabeth Hodson, Senior Dietitian
Leighton Hospital, Crewe

Vicky Johnson, Advanced Renal Dietitian, Wirral University Teaching Hospital NHS Foundation Trust

Maria Lee, Primary Care Dietitian
Wirral Primary Care Trust

Lowri Lloyd-Jones, Head of Primary Care Dietetic Services
Wirral Primary Care Trust

Helen Loughnane, Diabetes Specialist Dietitian, Royal Blackburn Hospital Blackburn

Jacqueline Love, Advanced Dietitian
Mersey Regional Burns Unit, Whiston Hospital, Merseyside

Nicky Mizen, Advanced Dietitian in Elderly Care
Wirral Hospital NHS Trust, Arrowe Park Hospital

Kathryn Morton, Dietetic Services Manager
Bolton Primary Care Trust

Solah Rasheed, Senior Dietitian
Ysbyty Gwynedd Hospital, Bangor

Emile Richman, Senior Dietitian
Royal Liverpool University Hospital, Liverpool

Julia Rosie, Senior Diabetes Dietitian
Wirral Hospital NHS Trust, Arrowe Park Hospital

Jacqui Ross, Dietetic Services Manager
North Cumbria Acute Hospitals NHS Trust, Cumberland Infirmary, Carlisle

Kathryn Simpson, Paediatric Dietitian
Leighton Hospital, Crewe

Wendy Swarbrick, Specialist Dietitian for Eating Disorders, East Lancashire
Primary Care Trust

Elizabeth Waters, Dietitian
Clatterbridge Centre for Oncology

Ruth Watling, Head of Dietetics
Royal Liverpool Children's NHS Trust, Liverpool

Claire Wesselingh, Diabetes Dietitian
Diabetes Centre, Whiston Hospital, Merseyside

Emma Whittle, Specialist Critical Care Dietitian, Mid Cheshire Hospitals NHS
Trust

Claire Wright, Senior Lecturer
University of Chester

Nirouz Zarroug, Senior Dietitian
Royal Liverpool University Hospital, Liverpool

The cases
(and contexts)

Case 1 Gillian Mercer

Diabetes

Study concepts: dietary compliance ■ lifestyle issues ■ management of a client with reduced access to local medical care

Study context: diabetes

Cases

Gillian Mercer was born in 1939 and for the past 18 years has lived in a small rural village about 1500 m above sea level, and 100 km east of Valencia in Spain. She owns an orchard and with her partner manages the day-to-day running of some 10 hectares of orange and lemon groves, walnut trees and a huge range of vegetables. What they do not eat themselves is sold to the local co-operative. Gillian also keeps a few goats and chickens. She and her partner enjoy a glass or two of Rioja each evening on their veranda, and Gillian is a heavy smoker.

Gillian is a Lancashire lass, and has returned to the UK for elective bowel surgery. She is diabetic and is taking metformin. She is now seven days post-op and is complaining bitterly about the hospital diet. She says it is tasteless, 'out of a packet or a tin', and is not what she is used to at all. She is used to tasty food and does not like the British hospital food (she usually cooks rice with a stock cube and loves home-cooked paella with fresh fish).

Gillian has lost 5 kg following surgery and her diabetes is not well controlled. Her usual dose of metformin at home is three tablets every day, but this has been restricted to two tablets as she is in hospital. Her blood sugar is described as high.

Gillian sees the dietitian and asks two main questions: 'Why can I not get powdered diabetic sugar "over here"?' and 'Why can I not have diabetic jam?'

Questions to consider

(1) The consultant physician asks you to review Mrs Mercer's diet. Discuss fully how you would approach this, explaining your rationale.
(2) Discuss and justify the nature of any dietary reinforcement you think might be appropriate.
(3) Discuss the issues for ongoing care in this case, given that the client has little or no access to medical services near her home.
(4) Explain any potential issues of compliance with dietary instruction.

Study questions

(1) Review the evidence base on which current dietary intervention of type 2 diabetes rests.

(2) Explain the short- and longer-term nutritional goals in the management of type 2 diabetes.

Case 2 The Odessa file

Renal disease, haemodialysis

Study concepts: dietary adherence to the unfamiliar UK diet ■ lifestyle issues ■ management of a client with impaired intellectual function and language issues ■ interpretation of clinical data

Study context: renal disease ■ haemodialysis

A 62-year-old man (67 kg; 175 m) from the Ukraine (Odessa, a village just north of Uman) is a refugee in the UK and is seeking British citizenship. He currently resides in a re-homing centre with fellow east European and Russian émigrés. He does not speak English and cannot read his first language well. He smokes 20 strong cigarettes/day and is unemployed. He is 'housed' with a cousin who speaks rather better English.

The man is admitted to the accident and emergency department of a large local teaching hospital with shortness of breath. He is discovered to have accelerated hypertension and has the following clinical chemistry:

Serum/plasma constituent	Result	Reference range
Albumin (g/l)	37	35–45
Creatinine (μmol/l)	1350	40–130
Haemoglobin (g/dl)	7.8	13.5–17.5 (male)
Phosphate (mmol/l)	2.97	0.8–1.4
Potassium (mmol/l)	3.8	3.5–5.0
Sodium (mmol/l)	133	135–150
Urea (mmol/l)	28.3	3.3–6.7

The man is considered to be a suitable candidate for peritoneal dialysis, but does not understand his medical problem and cannot learn the associated techniques of this mode of treatment. He is to start on hospital haemodialysis. His urine output is 500 ml/day. He is referred for dietary advice.

Questions to consider

(1) Comment on the clinical chemistry together with the other clinical information, indicating the priorities for medical and nutritional intervention.
(2) Calculate/estimate his major dietary requirements.
(3) Outline the major priorities for dietary intervention.
(4) Using key points only, indicate a possible outline for a therapeutic consultation.
(5) Discuss the patient's management in the context of the social issues.

Study questions

(1) Imagine you are to see this client for the first time. How would you prepare for a client who does not speak any English? What resources might be available to assist you?
(2) Review the treatment modalities of haemodialysis and peritoneal dialysis. Note the possible influences of these on the nutritional status of a patient.

Case 3 Darshan

Renal disease, peritoneal dialysis

Study concepts: interpretation of clinical data ■ therapeutic dietary issues in the context of a vegetarian lifestyle ■ management of aggressive nutritional support

Study context: renal disease ■ peritoneal dialysis

Darshan is a 51-year-old widowed Sikh (60 kg; 5 ft 8 in) who lives with his daughter and her large family. He has been feeling progressively unwell over the past few weeks and collapsed when he was tidying up the garden for the winter. He was taken to hospital by ambulance, accompanied by his daughter. He is a vegetarian, but will eat lamb on special occasions.

Darshan was admitted to the regional stroke unit and the diagnosis of a mild stroke was confirmed. His left-hand side has been affected. During the assessment, he was found to be hypertensive; an intra-venous pyelogram showed small, shrunken kidneys; a skeletal survey showed no evidence of osteoporosis. Some of his clinical chemistry lab results at admission were as shown overleaf.

Serum/plasma constituent	Result	Reference range
Alkaline phosphatase activity (u/l)	160	40–125
Creatinine (µmol/l)	1009	40–130
Phosphate (mmol/l)	3.01	0.8–1.4
Urea (mmol/l)	31.0	3.3–6.7

Peritoneal dialysis (PD) was started but was soon complicated by peritonitis (*Escherichia coli* and *Streptococcus* sp.).

Questions to consider

(1) Comment on the client's clinical data, indicating the significance of the clinical chemistry and how the data may inform management.
(2) Calculate the client's dietary requirements for energy and protein at baseline and during the period of peritonitis. Comment on the differences.
(3) Should the client have a subsequent stroke and the decision made to use a nasogastric feed, explain the factors to consider when calculating, delivering and monitoring the feed.

Study question

(1) Locate the current clinical guideline(s) in the management of this patient group and comment fully on the evidence underpinning the main nutritional prescription.

Case 4 Professor Plum

Renal disease, pre-dialysis

Study concepts: interpretation of clinical data ■ therapeutic dietary issues ■ justification of method of dietary assessment ■ formulation of a care plan

Study context: renal disease ■ pre-dialysis

Professor Plum is a 68-year-old history professor, in the UK on a sabbatical visit from Arizona, USA. Shortly after arrival in the UK, he began to feel nauseated and complained to a medical colleague of tiredness and a lack of energy. He is 176 m and weighs 96 kg.

He was referred for tests and a diagnosis of chronic renal failure was made. He is referred to the dietitian for dietary management. The following clinical data are available.

Serum/plasma constituent	Result	Reference range
Albumin (g/l)	40	35–45
Bicarbonate (mmol/l)	23	22–32
Calcium (mmol/l)	2.40	2.25–2.65
Creatinine (µmol/l)	637	40–130
Haemoglobin (g/dl)	8.1	13.5–17.5 (male)
Phosphate (mmol/l)	2.07	0.8–1.4
Potassium (mmol/l)	5.9	3.5–5.0
Sodium (mmol/l)	143	135–150
Urea (mmol/l)	15.3	3.3–6.7

Questions to consider

(1) Given the clinical information, what might be the client's likely symptomatology at diagnosis?
(2) Explain the clinical chemistry in relation to the decline in renal function.
(3) What might the management goals be in both the short and longer term?
(4) Explain, with justification, the dietary assessment likely to elicit the information that may be required to inform therapeutic dietary advice.
(5) Explain, with justification, the dietary advice that may be given.

Study questions

(1) Supposing a client such as Professor Plum remains nauseated for a number of days or weeks. What could be the dietary priorities in the short term and explain how the client might be managed as he progresses to a light hospital diet?
(2) What may be the main care implications for Professor Plum when he returns to the USA later in the year?
(3) Examine a relevant clinical guideline that relates to this client. Select any one recommendation for nutritional intervention (e.g. for protein/energy requirements) and study the evidence supporting the recommendation. Critically appraise the strength of the evidence.

Case 5 Annie
Renal disease, pre-dialysis

Study concepts: interpretation of clinical data ■ therapeutic dietary issues ■ justification of method of dietary assessment ■ possible decision to assist diet with artificial nutrition support

Study context: renal disease ■ pre-dialysis

Annie is an 82-year-old woman who lives alone with only Socrates (her cat) for company. She largely looks after herself, and although she owns her own house, the only real income she has is her state pension. She has contact with an estranged daughter-in-law who takes her shopping to a large out-of-town supermarket once every week. She is able to walk to the local mini-market when she has to, to buy her fresh food. She has a pint of whole milk delivered every other day. She has a small refrigerator.

Recently, Annie has become forgetful (neighbours report her leaving lights on) and the house has become tatty. She is generally not coping. Her height is currently 152 m and she weighs 43.5 kg. She was admitted to a rehabilitation and assessment ward where she reported a poor appetite with recent but modest weight loss. Creatinine clearance was assessed to be 4 ml/min. Bloods were taken and the following clinical data reported in her notes.

Serum/plasma constituent	Result	Reference range
Albumin (g/l)	30	35–45
Bicarbonate (mmol/l)	15	22–32
Calcium (mmol/l)	1.91	2.25–2.65
Creatinine (µmol/l)	430	40–130
Phosphate (mmol/l)	1.60	0.8–1.4
Potassium (mmol/l)	5.4	3.5–5.0
Sodium (mmol/l)	146	135–150
Urea (mmol/l)	18.0	3.3–6.7

Questions to consider

(1) Comment on the clinical data, explaining fully how these inform and influence the priorities for management.
(2) Describe and justify the possible approaches that may be used in the assessment of Annie's dietary intake.
(3) Calculate the dietary requirements for energy and protein and comment on the requirements for dietary intake of potassium and phosphorus.
(4) Assuming she is permitted to go home, justify the approach that may be taken with dietary management with reference to how Annie might achieve optimal dietary compliance.
(5) Discuss fully the discharge planning arrangements that may be considered appropriate.

Study question

(1) Using evidence to justify your answer, comment fully on the risk of malnutrition in a case like Annie, and discuss possible strategies to avoid this.

Case 6 Jon

Obesity

Study concepts: interpretation of dietary assessment ■ therapeutic dietary issues ■ justification of method of dietary and eating assessment ■ forming a clinical decision

Study context: obesity

Jon is 27 years of age, has a desk-bound job and currently weighs 155 kg and is 176 cm tall. He is single and a former professional cricketer. He now plays an occasional match for a local amateur club, but prefers instead to watch his extensive video collection of cricket matches from the comfort of his armchair.

At a recent friendly match he fell whilst bowling and twisted his left ankle. He had an X-ray at the local hospital. The radiology report read as follows:

Soft tissue swelling around lateral malleolus. No #. Old ankle injuries

Jon was prescribed ibuprofen by the nurse consultant in the accident and emergency department and referred to the dietitian for weight management dietary advice. The dietitian arranges to see him at a routine clinic and it transpires that he is a 'glutton' (self-confession and at history). He claims to eat a whole cooked chicken at a time for meals, or half a chicken if he isn't feeling hungry.

Questions to consider

(1) Justify the preferred method of dietary assessment that may be used at a first review of this client.
(2) Explain the concept of 'gluttony' and how this may affect construction of an intervention diet, dietary compliance and hence clinical outcome.
(3) Calculate the client's energy requirements using an evidence-based model of intervention practice.
(4) Translate this information to a diet sheet or other dietary education material, showing clearly how the intervention diet is constructed.
(5) Explain the approach that may be taken at interview and follow-up.

Study questions

(1) In the context of obesity, comment fully on the routine practice of classifying a client using BMI.

(2) Examine the evidence that correlates BMI with associated health risk and write an argument to use waist circumference to assess nutritional status.

Case 7 Mr Smart

Obesity, renal calculi

Study concepts: interpretation of descriptive information ■ dietary issues of quantitative and qualitative approaches ■ estimation of dietary energy requirements to induce weight loss.

Study context: obesity with renal calculi

Mr Smart is a 44-year-old marine engineer who works on a North Sea oil rig for periods of four to six weeks at a time. He has been complaining of an acute pain in his groin and failed a recent company medical. Following X-ray, blood and 24-hr urine investigations, a small kidney stone was detected. His blood work and data were normal, except for slightly raised levels of uric acid, serum cholesterol and triglycerides. His weight is stable (93 kg). He has a family history of renal reflux. He has been a heavy drinker and whilst his liver is predicted to be fatty (provisional diagnosis based on the slightly raised levels of serum cholesterol and triglycerides), liver function tests are relatively normal. He is 5 ft 11 in and does not exercise. He also has a Randall's plaque. He has been told not to return to work until his diet is managed. He is currently taking allopurinol.

The medical practitioner asks you to see Mr Smart. He requests a dietary investigation with a view to improving the client's diet. At review, the dietitian finds an erratic eating pattern characterised mainly by: nil for breakfast, a huge lunch consisting of sandwiches (eight slices of bread spread thickly with cheap margarine filled with meat) and a typical evening 'rig meal' of fry-ups and heavy puddings. He drinks only water throughout the day (about 600 ml in total) when he remembers.

Questions to consider

(1) Outline the dietary goals (short- and longer-term) for Mr Smart.
(2) Calculate his requirements for dietary energy, as a baseline for working towards an energy-deficit model of energy prescription.
(3) Estimate and justify his final dietary prescription for weight reduction, taking into account his activity level and required energy deficit to induce weight loss and maintenance.

(4) Prepare a model outline of his new diet using usual foods in standard portions.
(5) Account for any adjustments in the quality of his new diet in terms of renal stones (and control of symptoms) and preferred lipid biochemistry.

Study questions

(1) Study the prescribing criteria for allopurinol, and explain its use and mode of action.
(2) Consider and justify a prescription for physical activity to assist with weight loss, weight maintenance and general health improvement.

Case 8 Susan Ritzio
Ulcerative colitis

Study concepts: impact of diagnosis and surgical procedure on lifestyle ■ connection between symptoms and intervention advice ■ role of corticosteroids in disease management ■ short- and longer-term nutritional considerations

Study context: ulcerative colitis ■ surgical intervention

Susan Ritzio is a 28-year-old student teacher who was diagnosed just after her twentieth birthday as having ulcerative colitis. Her weight at diagnosis was 8.5 stone; she is 5 ft 9 in tall. Despite her low weight, she remains a competitive kick boxer.

Susan was admitted as an emergency with abdominal pain, rectal bleeding and colonic inertia, following an episode of *Campylobacter jejuni* infection. The decision was made to perform a laparoscopic total abdominal colectomy with j-pouch procedure. The patient remains on a small holding dose of prednisolone and is currently being treated for anaemia.

The colorectal surgeon told Susan to *go easy with food* during the postoperative period (six to eight weeks). The patient asks to see the dietitian to clarify the nature of specific food or drink to be concerned about, both in the short and longer term.

Questions to consider

(1) The patient requests to see you, the dietitian, to review what the surgeon meant by 'go easy with food'. Discuss fully how you might approach this consultation, explaining fully your rationale.

(2) Discuss the nature of any dietary instructions you think might be appropriate for a patient who has had laparoscopic total abdominal colectomy with j-pouch procedure.

(3) Discuss the issues for ongoing care in this case, given that the client has little or no access to medical services local to her home.

(4) Discuss any potential issues of compliance with dietary instruction.

Study questions

(1) Revisit the signs and symptoms that may be presented by a client with ulcerative colitis.

(2) Consider the signs and symptoms in relation to the surgeon's decision to perform the procedure.

(3) What might be the principal care themes in the peri- and post-operative period?

Case 9 Mr Rodger

Irritable bowel syndrome

Study concepts: lifestyle considerations of symptomatology ■ impact of lifestyle modification on symptoms ■ relationship between dietary behaviour and symptoms ■ controversy with regard to dietary intervention

Study context: irritable bowel syndrome

Mr Rodger is a junior partner in a large practice of solicitors and has suffered for some time from irritable bowel syndrome. His primary symptom is bloating, especially toward the end of the working day and into the evening, although he complains of generalised abdominal discomfort most of the time. He reports having to loosen his belt from time to time, to relieve some of the discomfort. He drives everywhere and does not devote time for exercise. He often pops in to a local wine bar for a snack on the way home from work; he pops into a take-away coffee shop on his way to work in the morning for a skinny cappuccino 'to go'. He lives alone and is no great lover of cooking. He buys ready-made food.

He mostly remains well and is keen to try changing his diet or lifestyle to reduce symptoms associated with bloating. He is health conscious, provided it takes little effort. He is referred to see the dietitian by the consultant gastroenterologist.

Questions to consider

(1) Prioritise the main issues that might inform the basis of an outpatient consultation.
(2) Discuss the symptomatology in relation to lifestyle issues presented in this case.
(3) Wrestle with the controversy surrounding dietary intervention for irritable bowel syndrome. In terms of dietary advice, what might be best practice for Mr Rodger?
(4) Consider Mr Rodger's typical dietary behaviour. Sketch out a likely framework of what you might include in a letter to the physician following the consultation.

Study questions

(1) Explore the range of dietary interventions that may be considered in formulating dietary advice for a client with irritable bowel syndrome. Given the evidence, map out a possible care plan for clients.
(2) Make the connection between dietary pattern and lifestyle issues that may exacerbate the symptoms presented in irritable bowel syndrome. Write a clear rationale for lifestyle advice for such clients.

Case 10 Pauline Trotter

Obesity, pharmacological management

Study concepts: management of long-standing obesity ■ lifestyle issues of clients ■ prescription/self-prescription of weight management drugs ■ management of secondary conditions

Study context: obesity ■ weight management

Pauline Trotter is a 42-year-old woman who works at a local high school dining facility. Her weight has gradually increased over the years and she is now beginning to have problems associated with long-standing obesity, including back pain and shortness of breath on exertion. She does very little in the way of exercise, and although she does not drive, she does not walk any further than she has to.

On a recent trip to the Philippines, Mrs Trotter bought some slimming pills at a clinic. She claims to have lost a significant amount of weight without really trying. On her return to the UK, she asked her GP to prescribe these pills to her. The GP does not think that she is a suitable candidate for the treatment and refers her to you for dietary reinforcement. You have seen her at clinic some years before, but without significant improvement in weight. She currently has a body mass index of $36\,kg/m^2$.

Questions to consider

(1) What might be the client's management goal(s) both in the short and longer terms?
(2) Discuss the client's likely motivation, given her eagerness to rely on pharmacological control of her condition.
(3) Map out for Mrs Trotter a possible diet and lifestyle plan, making a clear outline based on evidence-based dietary intervention best practice.

Study questions

(1) Consider the prescribing criteria that may help to inform the decision to prescribe pharmacological agents to assist with weight management.
(2) Outline the role of motivation in a client such as this and consider how this may have a positive impact in this case.
(3) Consider the key principles of motivational interviewing as it relates to therapeutic interaction with overweight/obese clients.
(4) Reflect on your ability to motivate a client. Draw up a personal plan for improvement/development based on comparing your skills with those you have mentioned in (3).

Case 11 Harriet Baker

Obesity, metabolic issues

Study concepts: managing obesity against a history of depressive illness ■ cyclical weight loss and regain ■ thyroid function complications ■ weight loss resistance ■ dietary compliance issues

Study context: obesity and weight management

Harriet Baker is obese (BMI $35\,kg/m^2$) and has been treated in the past for depression (tricyclic anti-depressant therapy), although she is not currently on medication. She has an under-active thyroid gland, for which she is currently prescribed thyroxine 100 mg/d; this allows her to be euthyroid. Her sleep pattern is disturbed (night phobia), for which she is taking promethazine. She also takes diazepam for spontaneous panic attacks.

Harriet presented at clinic with shortness of breath and that she feels zombie-like, has low self-esteem and is at least 3 stone heavier than she should or wants to be. She also complains that an old back injury is beginning to play up. She maintains that she cannot lose weight because of her metabolism. She has tried a high fat, low carbohydrate diet with moderate success, losing about a stone in weight, but could not maintain the diet. She has recently been prescribed a lipase inhibitor (orlistat) and has lost about 12 lb. In both instances she regained the weight. She is 62 years of age, lives on her own, with only her state pension to live on.

Questions to consider

(1)   Calculate a possible dietary energy prescription for Mrs Baker and map this against the typical daily pattern of foods that may be recommended to form the basis of her eating plan.
(2)   Imagine the first consultation: what might be the client's motivation and how might dietary adherence be encouraged? Indicate how one might assess the client's readiness to change her eating behaviour.
(3)   Apart from dietary changes, what other lifestyle changes might be appropriate?
(4)   She fails to attend a follow-up appointment but comes to a subsequent appointment having lost no weight. Discuss possible approaches that may be taken at the review appointment.

Study questions

(1)   Write down some prescribing information on lipase inhibitors as used to assist management of the obese client.
(2)   Enter the word 'depression' into a search engine on the Internet and make some informative notes from peer-reviewed websites on the pathology, treatment and implications for managing clients with this condition.

Case 12 Mr Cunningham

Functional dyspepsia, weight loss

Study concepts: short term management of acute weight loss ■ weight regain complicated by diarrhoea ■ drugs to control gastric motility ■ disturbance in fluid balance

Study context: functional dyspepsia ■ acute weight loss

Mr Cunningham is a 35-year-old oil refinery worker who has recently been on a short-term contract on an off-shore rig off the coast of Sweden. On his last night at sea, he began to feel unwell following a meal of Thai prawns. Since the episode of food poisoning, he has had frequent occurrences of diarrhoea and waves of sickness and continues to lose weight, going from 92 kg to 83 kg in a period of seven weeks.

On Mr Cunningham's return to the UK, he was examined by a general physician, who performed an upper gastrointestinal series of tests, using endoscopy. The examination showed mild inflammation in the body and fundus of the stomach. There was no evidence of *Helicobacter pylori* infection. The physician concluded that his problems were caused by functional dyspepsia (gastric dysmotility) and the patient was prescribed domperidone (10 mg three times daily).

Questions to consider

(1) Outline the management objectives for Mr Cunningham immediately following the diagnosis of food poisoning, assuming vomiting and diarrhoea are still prevalent and two of the key symptoms.

(2) How would the management change as the vomiting subsides and the pattern of diarrhoea changes from frequent daily episodes to intermittent weekly episodes?

(3) How might weight gain be achieved through conservative dietary measures, and over what term?

Study questions

(1) Explain the pathogenesis of *Helicobacter pylori* infection and why it was important to exclude this diagnosis in a client such as Mr Cunningham.

(2) Explain the mode of action of domperidone and why it might be appropriate to prescribe this drug in this case.

(3) Familiarise yourself with an upper gastrointestinal series of tests using endoscopy, as a tool to assist with arriving at a diagnosis.

Case 13 Mrs Rose Petroni

Obesity, infection, wound healing

Study concepts: post-surgical trauma and infection ■ fluid balance ■ nutritional intakes and wound healing ■ nutritional requirements influenced by presence of obesity and infection ■ anaemia

Study context: wound healing complicated by persistent infection ■ obesity

Mrs Rose Petroni is a 45-year-old overweight woman some four weeks post-abdominoplasty (fleur-de-lis procedure). Prior to surgery she was in excellent health, despite her obesity. She presented as a tanned and well-nourished woman, and she is very conscious of her well-groomed appearance. She has just returned from a trip to Japan, accompanying her husband on a business trip, and enjoyed a pearl diving holiday.

Mrs Petroni began to feel hot and sticky some 10 days post-operatively and was re-admitted for investigation of pyrexia. Following examination by the plastic surgeon, the abdominoplasty was found to be grossly infected. The wound was drained and then debrided. The patient's wound remained weepy for some time; her haemoglobin and potassium concentrations were low. She was given iron sulphate therapy. Her appetite was poor. She tested positive for *Staphylococcus aureus*. Her current weight is 75 kg and she is 5 ft 2 in tall.

Questions to consider

(1) Rose is an otherwise healthy, overweight person. What might be her diet priorities following a clean abdominal procedure?
(2) What are her primary treatment objectives now, following her re-admission to hospital?
(3) Explain the possible implications of low concentrations of haemoglobin and potassium and formulate a plan for dietary intervention to add to Question (2).
(4) Write some key points for improving her oral intake whilst in hospital.

Study questions

(1) Anaemia and appetite failure may be inter-related. Explain the likely connection between the two factors and discuss how improvement in iron status may improve spontaneous oral intake.
(2) Consult some recent research papers examining the positive influence of oral diet on wound healing outcome. Summarise the findings.
(3) What might be the impact on clinical management of using therapy such as iron supplements and antibiotics in a patient such as this?

Case 14 Linda Middlemiss
Arthralgia, food intolerance

Study concepts: food sensitivity ■ dietary assessment using a food and symptom record (diary) ■ evidence of impact of low allergen diet used in various conditions ■ managing erratic eating behaviour

Study context: arthralgia ■ food intolerance

Linda Middlemiss is a 53-year-old woman with a diagnosis of arthralgia. She has lupus and finds it very difficult to exercise. She continues to work from home where there is no stress, but she is concerned about her weight (currently 95 kg; height 160 cm) and presence of persistent constipation. She receives medication for heartburn and self-prescribes supplements of evening primrose oil.

The patient is concerned about health generally; her mother died from cancer of the bowel. She is a woman who reports extensive use and variety of foods in her diet, though she may eat erratically, depending on 'how the mood takes her'. She is an enthusiastic cook.

Linda is asked to keep a four-day diet diary to assist you with making a judgement about her dietary intake and subsequent intervention.

Questions to consider

(1) Comment fully on the primary diagnosis of arthralgia and note down key points (as bullets) evidencing aspects of diet that may be involved in managing the client.
(2) What might a diary tell you that might assist in coming to a decision about possible dietary intervention(s)?
(3) Are there any lifestyle issues associated with the patient that may be useful to consider in management?
(4) Assuming the client is managed jointly for obesity and arthralgia, are there similarities or differences in approach to food selection on the improved diet?

Study questions

(1) What is evening primrose oil, what are its 'claimed' properties and how is this form of complementary therapy reputed to benefit client groups at large?
(2) Note the major causes of constipation and explain the mechanisms involved.
(3) How may constipation be tackled by dietary means in clients unable to participate in physical activity or who have reduced mobility?
(4) How may an irregular eating pattern be tackled successfully in a therapeutic interview to result in regular eating (of a changed diet)?

Case 15 Josh Herriot

Coeliac disease, new diagnosis

Study concepts: dietary management of coeliac disease in differing contexts ■ the relationship between this disease and calcium status ■ delivering dietary advice at first and review consultations

Study context: newly diagnosed coeliac disease

Josh Herriot is a very pleasant 49-year-old farmer, who manages a large show herd of dairy cows in an isolated town in the Scottish Borders. He is a 'big lad' but has recently experienced weight loss and developed a change in bowel habit consistent with steatorrhoea. There is a strong family history of coeliac disease.

Following investigation, Josh's anti-endomysial antibodies are strongly positive, and a duodenal biopsy shows full (or 'flat') partial villous atrophy. A diagnosis of coeliac disease is confirmed. He presents to the dietitian for dietary advice.

Josh's one pastime is his love of the sea and he will soon be taking part in a tall ships' race, joining the crew on the *SS Kobenhaven*. It leaves for a four to six weeks' race around the British Isles. He is keen to have his diet sorted out before then.

Questions to consider

(1) Outline Josh's diet priorities given his daily lifestyle and social context.
(2) Take a few moments to consider the structure of a potential therapeutic interview. Determine Josh's therapeutic goals and how the dietitian can work towards achieving them at both his first visit to clinic and his first annual review appointment.
(3) Study a clinical guideline for coeliac disease that includes reference to improving calcium status of patients. Draw up a 'bone friendly' diet sheet that will assist Josh in achieving this clinical outcome.
(4) What practical solutions might be given to this client for managing his diet at home on the farm and 'at sea'?

Study questions

(1) Make some informative notes on the features of undiagnosed coeliac disease and how these relate to clinical management priorities to improve nutritional status.
(2) There are a number of key age categories of clients presenting with coeliac disease. List these and indicate any specific approaches or practical management issues that are age-specific.

Case 16 Carly Carpenter

Disordered eating in adulthood

Study concepts: eating disorders complicated by depression and family struggles ■ eating swings related to heavy menstrual periods

Study context: disordered eating in adulthood

Carly Carpenter is a 30-year-old woman with a history of bulimic eating disorder since aged 12 years. She claims that her eating patterns arise from depression and family pressures (she comes from a broken home, she is now a lone parent and has responsibility for a chronically ill mother). Her son is 1 year old and she has returned to work as a part-time pharmacy representative.

Carly's diet pattern is erratic and her eating behaviour strongly associated with her moods and whether or not she is working. She is currently 100 kg (height 1.64 m). She has a bingeing pattern in the early evening (3/7) consisting of three chocolate bars, six cream cakes, one packet of biscuits (chocolate digestives are her favourite) and a whole fruitcake, in addition to her usual diet. She does not presently have a vomiting phase, but will try to follow bingeing sessions with a trip to the gym. She adores gin and tonic, and may have several drinks most evenings. Occasionally she will raid the refrigerator in the middle of the night. She is constantly tired and referred to the dietitian by the consultant psychiatrist.

Questions to consider

(1) Discuss what might be the plan for the first outpatient consultation with Carly, explaining clearly the key steps in the therapeutic interview.
(2) List the short- and longer-term goals for the client, taking into account that she may be resistant to changing her lifestyle.
(3) The client reports that she has particularly painful periods and this usually coincides with a huge increase in consumption of sweet foods. What specific advice might be given to help resolve her cyclical cravings?

Study questions

(1) Comment fully on the likely adherence with dietary and lifestyle intervention and on the likelihood of achieving good clinical outcome.
(2) Make a few notes on the pathology and development of bulimic eating disorder in our society today.
(3) Research the evidence that implicates eating behaviour in later life being attributed to eating patterns in early life. Summarise these.
(4) Consider the management of a client with bulimic eating disorder. What particular clinical skills might be developed to assist in any dietary intervention?

Case 17 Mr Tony Marshall

Obesity, renal calculi

Study concepts: lifestyle issues associated with management of renal calculi

Study context: kidney stones ■ obesity

Mr Tony Marshall has a history of kidney stones and recently failed a medical routinely performed by the occupational health department. He has raised levels of uric acid and may have a small renal stone currently. He has recently celebrated his fiftieth birthday with family and friends. He is a long-haul airline pilot.

Tony has been a heavy drinker in the past and LFTs have revealed a somewhat damaged liver. He has been trying to self-limit his calcium intake with respect to his kidney stones as a result of going on a website he found on the Internet. He is currently 103 kg (5 ft 11 in). He likes his food, confesses to eating very large portions, especially of salty/high fat foods and snacks and he reports that his favourite foods include cheddar cheese, milk (full fat) and pizzas. He is referred to the dietitian.

Questions to consider

(1) Explain what the therapeutic plan might be for Mr Marshall in managing his weight.
(2) Comment fully on how his occupation and love of food might complicate dietary adherence.
(3) Explain the extent to which it may be useful to consider managing his history of kidney stones by diet and/or lifestyle.
(4) Assuming intervention takes the form of general dietary advice, what particular aspects of the information may be important, and why?
(5) Assume he comes back to clinic for review, say in eight weeks, and has lost 5 kg. Consider the key points that may be useful to consider at the review appointment interview.

Study questions

(1) Review the evidence implicating diet and lifestyle in the risk associated with development of renal calculi. Comment on the weight of evidence and how this may affect diet and lifestyle priorities in this case.
(2) Comment fully on the extent to which faulty snacking behaviour may be associated with the onset of overweight and obesity.
(3) Consider the role of both intake of fluid and NSPs in the therapeutic management of this case. What might be their role in long-term management?

Case 18 Carrie West

Bulimia nervosa

Study concepts: binge-eating behaviour in social context, managing diet in seclusion ■ managing a change in eating behaviour ■ selection of appropriate means of dietary assessment

Study context: bulimia nervosa

Carrie West is a 17-year-old schoolgirl who does some part-time modelling work for a photographic agency. She is a striking looking girl and has a history of bulimic eating behaviour. She appears to eat very little (an apple during the day, following by a huge meal in the evening, which she has with her family). She self-induces vomiting following the evening meal. Presently she does not look overly thin but she is a very anxious girl and probably has some underlying depressive illness. She is not on anti-depressive medication.

Carrie's parents are divorced and she lives with both families. She is keen to seek dietary advice and she knows that her binge/eating behaviour is far from normal. She arrives at the outpatient clinic with an older relative (not a parent). Her dietary intake is assessed by the dietitian and it is estimated that she consumes almost all of her dietary energy at the single evening meal (800–1000 kcal/d).

Questions to consider

(1) Explain the thinking behind the form of dietary assessment that may be chosen for this client and why.
(2) List the treatment goals for Carrie and consider fully the steps which may be taken to take the client towards good clinical outcome(s).
(3) Carrie clearly does not want her parents to know her diagnosis or treatment plan. Comment on this feature of her history and whether you think this may have a bearing on the treatment or outcome.
(4) How might one approach the issue of vomiting (bingeing) behaviour, in the context of a dietetic consultation?

Study questions

(1) Consider fully the epidemiology associated with the development of a bulimic eating disorder and the extent to which blame might be attributed to peer pressure.
(2) Classify what might be known or described as 'normal eating', in terms of the number and size of eating occasions per day and try to distinguish between normal and unusual eating behaviours.
(3) Obtain copies of tools (e.g. questionnaires) that attempt to diagnose or classify eating behaviour(s). Describe these and comment fully on their likely validity and sensitivity.

Case 19 Holly Shakespeare

Obesity, polycystic ovarian syndrome

Study concepts: weight management in polycystic ovarian syndrome ■ loss of incentive to maintain weight loss progress

Study context: polycystic ovarian syndrome ■ obesity

Holly Shakespeare is a 24-year-old librarian with a nine-month history of amenorrhoea since stopping the combined contraceptive pill. She presented herself at the gynaecology outpatient clinic somewhat anxious about her irregular periods, and more especially because of accelerated growth in facial hair. She smokes 25 cigarettes a day and has recently gained about 20 kg in weight, taking her into the obese category of BMI.

A pelvic examination was normal; she had normal serum concentrations of follicle-stimulating hormone and prolactin. Her testosterone level, however, was 3.1 nmol/l, which is slightly elevated. A diagnosis of polycystic ovarian syndrome was made and the gynaecologist is convinced that weight loss would allow her to ovulate and her periods to become regular.

The dietitian sees her and advises on appropriate lifestyle changes. An energy-deficit eating plan is commenced, calculated from her current weight and exercise output. She reports that she is 'not big on fruit and vegetables'. She comes back to clinic to be reviewed on two occasions, and loses 10% of total body weight over a span of 16 weeks. She is delighted, but more especially as her periods have started again.

Questions to consider

(1) What might be the particular difficulties of managing a patient with obesity and polycystic ovarian syndrome?

(2) Are there any specific aspects of a therapeutic interview that require particular focus for a client of this type?

(3) Assuming Holly continues to be reviewed, and her weight begins to increase, what approaches might be employed to encourage further weight loss and maintenance?

Study questions

(1) Consider in some depth the features and underlying pathology of polycystic ovarian syndrome and make a few helpful notes.

(2) Write a short dietary checklist, consisting of useful goals, to assist clients with making good diet and lifestyle choices to better manage this condition.

Case 20 Barry Morgan
Post-surgical weight loss, appetite failure

Study concepts: managing food and drink intake during appetite failure ■ estimating nutritional requirements in a post-surgical patient

Study context: post-surgical weight loss ■ surgical trauma ■ appetite failure

Barry Morgan is a middle-aged man who was recently admitted for a post-anterior resection of colon, following excision of a T2 tumour. The nutritional screening tool has revealed a high score indicating significant nutritional risk.

Barry is 5 ft 7 in tall and weighs 76.2 kg. His pre-operative weight was 81.2 kg, and he is now nine days post-op. A short course nasogastric feed (seven days) was established, essentially because of nausea and poor oral intake. This has now been withdrawn but the patient still has persistent nausea. He remains on an intra-venous dextrose drip. Whilst on the ward, a nurse passes you in the corridor and comments 'you'll have to see Mr Morgan – he's not eating a thing and his albumins are in his boots!'. The patient's notes are checked and it is confirmed that his serum albumin concentration is low (<28 g/l) and there is general concern about his oral intake.

The patient is seen by the dietitian and it is noted that his spontaneous appetite remains poor, some 48 hours following feed withdrawal. You estimate that his total intake amounts to about 300 kcal/d. He is not a great lover of sweet foods.

Questions to consider

(1) List some points of the client's main nutritional goals, stating clearly what might be his clinical priorities.
(2) Estimate his main nutritional requirements using the limited clinical data revealed in the case.
(3) Assuming his oral hospital diet intake increases to provide 700 kcal and 30 g protein/d, outline the practical measures that may assist Mr Morgan in achieving optimal nutritional intake.
(4) Comment on the route of patient referral in this case.

Study questions

(1) Draw up some helpful guidelines to increase oral intake for a group of clients who are nauseous.
(2) Outline the processes that may be involved in coping strategically with a client who refuses to consume a specific energy-dense dietary supplement.
(3) Consider techniques that may be used in the monitoring of a client's food and drink intake and comment on their ability to inform decisions about feeding a client.
(4) Comment fully on the value of serum albumin concentration as a parameter indicating nutritional status.
(5) Comment briefly on tumour classification as a means of describing stage of disease, likely prognosis and indication for nutritional intervention.

Case 21 Rayan Hussein

Iron-deficiency anaemia, ethnic diet

Study concepts: dietary exploration ■ dietary assessment methodology ■ communication barrier with a client

Study context: possible iron and folic acid deficiency anaemia in an ethnic minority client

Rayan Hussein is a 33-year-old woman from northern Pakistan. She is a software engineer and is married with non-identical twins aged 3 years. She has been living in Belfast for about a year and prior to this she lived in the United States. She has recently been referred to the gastrointestinal unit with symptoms of abdominal discomfort. She has had a full gastrointestinal series (upper and lower) of tests with no apparent significant pathology detected. She has constipation and unexplained folic acid and iron deficiency that arouses suspicion that her diet may be at fault. She weighs 57.3 kg and has a BMI of 19 kg/m². She reports experiencing less abdominal discomfort on a self-inflicted low fat diet. She claims to eat fruit and vegetables and she denies weight loss. She is currently prescribed 200 mg ferrous sulphate and 5 mg folic acid daily, which is correcting her anaemia. She is to continue this until reviewed by the consultant and dietitian.

Rayan comes to clinic with a companion. The interview is complicated, not because of the standard of her English, but because she seems reluctant to speak at all. Her diet is to some extent Westernised, but she continues to rely as much as possible, on familiar and traditional foods.

Questions to consider

(1) Outline the possible structure of the outpatient consultation, explaining what might be achieved during the session.

(2) Indicate, with reasons, the methodology of the dietary assessment, including the particular nutrients that may be useful to investigate.

(3) Indicate what homework might be done in advance of the consultation, in preparation for meeting the client.

(4) Invent some possible marginal values of dietary intake arising from a virtual assessment of this client. Draft a letter to the referring consultant using these data to explain your findings in relation to nutritional status and likely dietary fault(s).

Study questions

(1) Review the traditional diet of Rayan's ethnic minority group and indicate potential nutritional problems associated with retaining the dietary pattern in the UK.

(2) How might you encourage a client to speak at a consultation, when the client clearly does not want to engage in conversation?

(3) What particular approaches may be employed when a client clearly demonstrates undue dietary restraint that may be related to detriment of nutritional quality of the intake?

Case 22 Peggy

Dementia

Study concepts: management of diet associated with dementia ■ bizarre dietary behaviour ■ movement from independent eating to eating dependency

Study context: diet in dementia

Peggy is a 65-year-old widow who has Alzheimer's disease. She has had progressive memory loss over the past few years and her behaviour is becoming tiresome for her daughter with whom she has been living for the past 12 months. Her vocabulary is extremely limited; for the most part she remains unintelligible and is becoming increasingly frustrated.

Peggy has started to rummage in chests of drawers, pilfer food from the refrigerator, and hides food in clothing and cupboards. She has also begun to soil herself at toilet. She is underweight and is continuing to lose weight. She is becoming a very dependent eater and much prefers sweet foods, especially chocolate cake. She does not sleep well, and despite going to bed early, she frequently gets up at night to prowl. She attends a day centre 09.30–15.30 hours twice each week.

Peggy was admitted to hospital for one week's respite care to give her daughter a well-earned break but has been kept in hospital for an assessment. She is referred for dietetic assessment.

Questions to consider

(1) What kind of dietary and nutritional assessment might be most appropriate for Peggy, and why? Outline the questions that may be posed to her daughter.

(2) Give an explicit account of a typical care plan for the ongoing assess-ment whilst in hospital, including the dietary goals.

(3) What might be her longer-term dietary goals as she returns home to resume living with her daughter? How might these be achieved?

(4) Discuss the possible nutritional care plan that may be proposed should the decision be made to move Peggy into permanent residential care.

Study questions

(1) Consider fully the diagnostic criteria, pattern and pathology of this disease, paying particular focus to the timescale and progression of the condition.

(2) What is the current thinking of managing the condition pharmacologi-cally? Describe the clinical guideline relating to this group of clients and consider how a care home might assist in the delivery of this guideline for this group of patients.

Case 23 Cain

Cerebral palsy

Study concepts: management of diet in a child with difficult eating and intellectual issues ■ multi-disciplinary care ■ social issues associated with eating

Study context: diet in cerebral palsy

Cain is an 8-year-old child who has cerebral palsy. His intelligence quotient (IQ) is at the lower end of normal and although his speech is slurred, he communicates well, if slowly. He rocks continually, backwards and forwards.

Cain was born six weeks before term and has never managed to achieve the fiftieth centile for weight. He currently has a BMI of 15 kg/m^2 and has some difficulty walking. He also has an upper respiratory tract infection.

Cain's mother has become exasperated with her son's behaviour and most meal times are reported as a battleground. Completion of a meal may take as much as two hours. Cain has poor lip seal and mouth closure and often aspirates during feeding. Consequently, meal times are messy. He has an older sister who helps with meals and general supervision.

Questions to consider

(1) Highlight the aspects of Cain's history that may affect his nutritional status and indicate how these might be tackled, and by whom, to work towards a better plane of nutrition.

(2) Prioritise nutritional care for Cain in terms of short- and longer-term goals.

(3) The mother is especially concerned about his weight. What particular tips might you give her to encourage catch-up weight?

(4) What might be the implications of the history for other members of the MDT?

Study questions

(1) Consider fully the presenting features of cerebral palsy, noting especially the care implications for nutritional status.

(2) Discuss the measures that may be taken to monitor growth in a child with cerebral palsy.

(3) Inspect a normal child's developmental map noting landmarks for speech and socialisation. How does this compare in a child with cerebral palsy?

Case 24 Abel

Down's syndrome

Study concepts: management of Down's syndrome ■ messy dietary behaviour ■ monitoring a child's weight pattern ■ function of a growth (weight) chart and interpretation of data

Study context: diet in a child with Down's syndrome

Abel is a 10-year-old child who has Down's syndrome. There were no birth difficulties and he was born slightly over term. He is described in notes as having a good weight.

Abel is an affectionate, cheerful and friendly boy with an intelligence quotient (IQ) of only 60 points and goes to a specialist school. He is relatively articulate, but his speech is slightly sluggish. He has hypotonia, and his social skills at the meal table are a constant source of frustration for his family. He dribbles, although he is a relatively independent eater. He is a mouth breather. He is currently quite well although he suffers from regular appearance of abscesses in the mouth.

Questions to consider

(1)   Abel presents with a number of fairly typical features of Down's syndrome. Indicate how these may have an impact on achieving a good clinical outcome in terms of nutrition. Propose a communication strategy.

(2)   Construct a nutritional care plan for Abel.

(3)   Consider the issues that may positively influence dietary intake in this case and the personnel or family members that may enable this.

(4)   How might one encourage Abel to become more aware of his diet?

Study questions

(1)   Describe the features of a growth chart and explain these in relation to monitoring a child's growth.

(2)   Using the growth chart (for weight) in Figure 2, compare and contrast Abel with Cain (the previous case) in terms of baseline weight, nutritional status and longer-term goals. Plot the weight parameters (you might want to copy the chart or obtain your own to complete your answer) and discuss the plots in relation to expected patterns of growth in normal children. Explain any significant landmarks in weight pattern and try to relate this to possible pathological features of the conditions. Weight parameters are as follows:

Cain	Abel
2.85 kg (birth)	17 kg (age 2 years)
15 kg (age 2 years)	19 kg (age 4 years)
15 kg (age 4 years)	20 kg (age 6 years)
14.5 kg (age 6 years)	22 kg (age 8 years)
15.5 kg (age 8 years)	23 kg (age 10 years)

(3)   Find a Down's-specific growth chart. How does this differ from normal growth charts, and indicate any differences when using a growth chart such as this with a specific population of children. It may be useful to plot Abel's parameters on this to illustrate your answer.

2 to 20 years: Boys

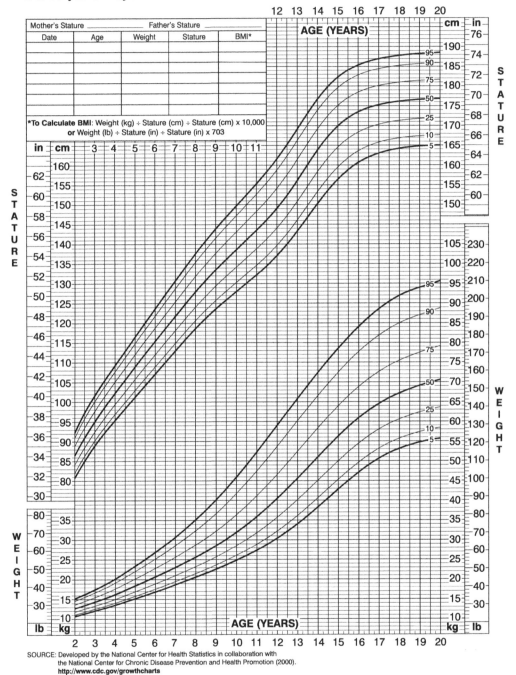

SOURCE: Developed by the National Center for Health Statistics in collaboration with
the National Center for Chronic Disease Prevention and Health Promotion (2000).
http://www.cdc.gov/growthcharts

Figure 2 Sample growth chart (5–18 years).

Case 25 Lucinda Smythe

Reactive hypoglycaemia

Study concepts: management of erratic eating and social behaviour ▪ diet and lifestyle intervention

Study context: reactive hypoglycaemia

Cases

Lucinda Smythe is a keen events woman. She has two horses: a novice (4 years) and a teenager. She leads an active life, and she has a husband and a 3-year-old daughter.

Lucinda's day starts at 06.00 hours when she snatches a slice of toast sometimes before driving to the stable to groom and clean up after her horses. She drives back to her home to get her daughter ready for nursery. She sits with her daughter at the breakfast table and has a cup of coffee with skimmed milk and sugar. Her husband looks after himself. She drives to work (a desk job) via the nursery, where she stays until 17.00 hours. She collects her daughter on the way home and she makes her a light tea (from which she may snack from) before visiting her horses again. Supper is usually eaten on her lap with a large glass of red wine.

Every time Lucinda drinks coffee she feels jittery. Sometimes her vision is blurred when driving and she often feels light-headed, particularly during competitions. Her blood sugar is almost always 3–4 mmol/l when tested, and her glucose tolerance tests are always in the normal range. Her diagnosis is reactive hypoglycaemia and she is referred for dietary management.

Questions to consider

(1) What kind of dietary assessment would you conduct, and why?
(2) Lucinda's dietary assessment reveals an erratic eating pattern. She prefers snack foods to proper meals. She does not like wholemeal or starchy foods (she believes them to be fattening and cannot afford to put on weight approaching competitions). She adores chocolate and sweet foods.
(3) Plan her diet and lifestyle intervention, with justification of the key points.

Study questions

(1) Explore the main metabolic aspects of the diagnosis and explain these to a learning partner.

(2) Consider the dietary factors that may assist in managing blood glucose control.

Case 26 Mrs Jolly

Type 2 diabetes

Study concepts: moving a client from a strict diet to evidence-based management ■ influencing dietary change using dietary reinforcement ■ diet and lifestyle interventions ■ methods of dietary education ■ the construct of a therapeutic interview

Study context: type 2 diabetes

Mrs Jolly is a slightly overweight woman who had been celebrating her golden wedding anniversary with her husband on board a cruise ship in the Mediterranean. As the holiday progressed, she began to feel more and more poorly, but put it down to finding her sea-legs and general excitement.

As guests of the captain at his table one evening, Mrs Jolly fainted and was taken to see the ship's doctor in the sickbay. After taking a brief history, the doctor concluded that she had diabetes. Later in the cruise, the ship's nurse instructed her on a formal low carbohydrate diet (about 140 g carbohydrate/d) based on a carbohydrate exchange system.

On returning home to her Welsh mining village, Mrs Jolly saw her family doctor who suspected that the diet she received on board ship was at best strict. He referred her on for specialist diet and lifestyle advice.

Questions to consider

(1) Discuss the ethics of the basis of the ship's diet.
(2) Explain and justify the approach that may be used with Mrs Jolly at the clinic.
(3) Compare the ship's diet with the clinic diet and explain fully the contrast, in terms of evidence-based nutrition intervention.
(4) Discuss the additional lifestyle interventions that may be beneficial in this case.

Study questions

(1) Consider the shape of an outpatient consultation interview with regard to intervention for a client with type 2 diabetes. Outline the possible

key landmarks for an interview, and state the relative importance of each step.

(2)   What particular skills might need to be taught to a newly-diagnosed diabetic client at first and reviewed at outpatient appointments?

(3)   Obtain a copy of any example of dietary education literature that may be used during the instruction of a diabetic client, and explain to your learning partner the principles on which it is based.

Case 27   Cordelia

Irritable bowel syndrome

Study concepts: using a diet diary to prioritise diet and lifestyle intervention recommendations

Study context: diet diary in a client with irritable bowel syndrome

Cordelia is an agony aunt who has a wide circle of friends. She flits from one social engagement to another, and she frequently misses meals and often rushes or bolts down her food. She is a little underweight and complains of abdominal bloating and flatulence. She reports having to loosen her belt during the course of her evening meal because of a swollen stomach. She is reluctant to talk about her age.

Cordelia's bowel habits are sporadic and fluctuate between constipation and diarrhoea. She complains of incomplete evacuation of her bowels and has spotted the passage of slimy stools that she sometimes has to pass with great urgency. She frequently holidays in her villa on the Costa Blanca where her general condition improves. However, she has recently returned from a rafting holiday in Egypt where she picked up a gastrointestinal infection. She is referred for dietary advice.

Question to consider

(1)   Following the diagnosis of irritable bowel syndrome, the client sends you a diet diary (together with a symptom record). Symptoms are quite non-specific and inconsistent for the period of four days' records, except that bloating continued throughout the evening. Study the intake, in the context of the history, and make considered diet and lifestyle recommendations. A typical day's intake is as follows:

Breakfast (09.00 hours)
2 cigarettes and a mug of strong black coffee with sugar (2 teaspoons)

Cases

Lunch (14.00 hours)
A salad Nicoise with two wedges of garlic bread and a glass of chilled Chianti

Evening meal (22.30 hours)
Bowl of minestrone soup
Lasagne (in a box, suitable for a microwave oven)
Green salad, French dressing and a few olives
Crème caramel with double cream
Strong black coffee with sugar
2 glasses of red wine whilst writing a column for next week's deadline

Nightcap
A glass of brandy, and a cigarette

Case 28 Josh

Human immunodeficiency virus (HIV)

Study concepts: effect of disease pattern on nutritional status ■ principles of dietary education ■ management of weight loss ■ methods of evaluation of dietary outcomes

Study context: diet in HIV infection

Josh is a 31-year-old hospital porter. He lives with his partner in a small flat near the hospital. He was found to be HIV positive following a short period of flu-like illness in 2001. He pays a lot of attention to his general health, and takes supplements, evening primrose oil and gingko biloba. He is also a keen runner.

Josh has started to feel a little tired and weak; he has become snappy and irritable. He complains of a dry, rough mouth and has developed watery diarrhoea which he voids about six times a day. He has night sweats and fever. He has virtually no appetite and the small amount of food that he does consume makes him feel sick.

Josh has lost about 5 kg in weight over the past four weeks. At clinic today he was told he had developed cryptosporidiosis infection. The doctor also told him to pay more attention to his diet. He refers him for dietary advice. He is 181 cm tall (61 kg) and has a CD4 count of 190.

Questions to consider

(1) Explain the significance of the signs and symptoms in the context of Josh's worsening nutritional status. What does a CD4 count tell us?
(2) Formulate the nutritional goals that may be appropriate for Josh and explain and justify the approach that may be taken at clinic.

(3)   Draw up a simple diet check list designed to encourage individuals with this diagnosis to improve their energy intake.

(4)   Decide on possible methods to evaluate progress towards improvement made on diet and nutritional status as Josh returns to clinic for review appointments.

Study questions

(1)   Consider the main impact on nutritional status made by the disease.

(2)   Examine the drugs that might be used to assist a client with HIV infection and the possible effects of these on nutritional status.

(3)   Consider any advice that may be given to a client, in terms of personal hygiene, and draw up a simple guide for use as an adjunct to diet information.

Case 29 Murdo MacKenzie
Cardiovascular and colorectal cancer risk

Study concepts: assessment of colorectal cancer and cardiovascular risk ■ consideration of specific dietary components in context ■ diet and lifestyle modifications

Study context: diet and behaviour modifications in relation to cardiovascular and colorectal cancer risk

Murdo MacKenzie is a former prop-forward rugby player and as he approaches 45 years of age he is carrying more weight than he used to during his playing days. He is based in the Highlands of Scotland where he has a responsible, but desk-bound job. He travels for his company on a regular basis within the UK, and on a recent trip to Glasgow, he went for a health scan. He is a little pre-occupied with the recent death of his brother because of colorectal cancer.

The assessment suggests that Mr MacKenzie should indeed think about losing some weight (he is currently 120 kg and 6 ft tall), and in addition he should do something to manage his cholesterol concentration (serum value on a fasting blood sample was 6.5 mmol/l). Bone density parameters are at the lower end of normal.

He approaches the dietitian for dietary advice. At interview, it is revealed that he is a hearty eater, but prefers meat to anything else. Indeed, much of his spare time is spent shooting with friends. His freezer is full of game, including snipe, venison, duck and partridge. After the shoot, he joins his friends for long sessions (eating and drinking) in the local hotel.

Questions to consider

(1) Explain what might be a reasonable approach to take in making diet and lifestyle modifications for this client?
(2) Assuming his diet consists predominantly of meat (2 meals/d containing 200 g meat), how might an attempt be made to bring this into line with more modest recommendations?
(3) Explain how you might tackle borderline bone density parameters.

Study questions

(1) Consider the evidence that implicates diet with colon cancer and attempt to ascribe the risk associated with Mr MacKenzie's diet and lifestyle.
(2) Compare and contrast the compositional details (qualitative and quantitative) of game foods compared with more usual meat sources and assess the likely impact of game foods in relation to cardiovascular health.
(3) Comment on the likely adherence to diet and lifestyle change in a client such as Mr MacKenzie.

Case 30 Anna Walker

Bone health

Study concepts: assessment of calcium status of a diet ■ diet and lifestyle modifications of a diet in relation to improving calcium status.

Study context: assessment of dietary calcium intake ■ bone health

Anna Walker has just had her fortieth birthday party. She presented some three years ago with cancer in the left breast and underwent a wide local excision followed by a right mastectomy at the end of last year with adjuvant chemotherapy. At the beginning of this year she has had a laparoscopic oophorectomy. A baseline bone density scan was carried out which was satisfactory but a subsequent scan has revealed a reduction in bone density of some 7.4%. She has been advised to increase her dietary calcium intake following completion of a routine calcium intake questionnaire carried out by the Osteoporosis Service. She is currently taking Adcal (a calcium supplement).

Anna is referred to you to assess her calcium intake.

Questions to consider

(1) Explain the possible influences of oophorectomy on bone status of a female client.

(2) Discuss how you would assess calcium intake and justify fully the method you recommend.

(3) Comment on the other nutrients that you may be interested in exploring in relation to those that may affect calcium status.

(4) Design a 'bone-friendly' information leaflet for this client group, highlighting key points and justifying their inclusion.

Study questions

(1) Apart from the client context in this case, indicate the population groups at greatest risk of calcium depletion.

(2) Indicate the main sources of dietary calcium, and classify these into groups relative to the calcium content (e.g. good sources, poor sources) and typical amounts eaten.

(3) Design a food frequency questionnaire to explore calcium content of a dietary intake.

Case 31 Shirley Stringfellow

Angioedema, salicylate exposure

Study concepts: assessment of diet in relation to likely dietary salicylate load ■ dietary intervention using salicylate-free dietary information

Study context: reducing dietary exposure to salicylates

Shirley Stringfellow is a 40-year-old mother of five. She is of normal weight with a very red face (angioedema) and has asthma. She complains of having little energy most of the time and that family stress is the trigger to her symptoms (she has three step-children from her husband's previous marriage, and is struggling with her financial affairs). Her acute symptoms are swelling of the lips and tongue and respiratory distress, which are related to her dietary pattern. Symptoms can arise 20 minutes after eating. A glass of red or white wine exacerbates her asthma. She has long-standing constipation.

Shirley is currently on very high doses of anti-histamines but the plan is to reduce these when a salicylate-free diet is implemented and well established. There is little doubt that she is sensitive to aspirin.

Questions to consider

(1) Discuss the type of dietary assessment that may be conducted in this case to assess likely risk of exposure to salicylate and aspirin.

(2) Construct a simple, but explicit dietary information pamphlet to indicate the likely major areas of dietary manipulation that may reduce risk of triggering a reaction.

(3) Outline the other lifestyle changes that may assist in reducing exposure to salicylates and derivatives.

(4) Consider the practical advice that may assist the client in making appropriate food choices.

Study questions

(1) Discuss the extent to which you think food labels may assist a client in making informed food choices with regard to additive/preservative composition.

(2) Assuming that the client was subsequently proved to be sensitive to benzoic acid, outline the additional dietary restrictions that may assist control of the angioedema.

(3) Discuss the impact of stress on nutritional status and the likely bearing that it may have in this case.

Case 32 Family tree
Diet and lifestyle change over time

Study concepts: assessment of diet and historical dietary and lifestyle issues using an interviewing technique and checklist ■ comparison of intakes and relationship with dietary exposure and dietary choices over a family timeline

Study context: assessment of diet by dietary recall and reporting

Dietary choices are in part affected by society, culture, peer pressure and social identity. With each passing generation, there are concerns about nutritional intakes and lifestyle pressures that may have implications for population interventions so that health risk can be minimised. It is therefore interesting to compare longitudinal dietary and lifestyle information from family members to assess relative risk in relation to social changes over time.

Study questions

(1)   Construct a family tree using yourself and siblings as the starting point and trace your family up through your mother or father (and their siblings); and their mothers and fathers (and siblings) and so on, until you reach the generation where a last family member is alive. This might be, for example, your grandmother/father, or great grandmother/ father.

(2)   Select one family member from each generation (or more if you wish) from whom you can obtain diet and lifestyle information. This will depend on access to family members or their ability to communicate information to you.

(3)   Design a list of questions (or checklist) that may assist you to make judgements about the diet and lifestyle of a generation that might allow you to piece together factual and longitudinal information.

(4)   Deliver the questions to one or more family members from each generation. What conclusions can you draw about dietary intake and lifestyle in a family down through the generations?

Case 33 *RMS Titanic*
Dietary judgement of menus

Study concepts: assessment of diet using a snapshot technique ■ comparison of intakes between socio-economic grouping ■ relationship between dietary exposure and likely health risk

Study context: assessment of diet by eyeballing menus

The ability to make informed assumptions about dietary composition is part of everyday practice for a dietitian. As dietary assessment methodology becomes necessarily quick, given the caseloads carried by many dietitians, it becomes essential to be able to make rapid, but nevertheless informed, judgements about diet and/or lifestyle.

As therapeutic interviews usually generate information about meal compositions and food items included in a daily intake (a day's menu), a dietitian may be faced with making broad assumptions based on a few key dietary items. Dietitians are also called to inspect hospital or care home menus, for example, and simply eyeball them for a crude idea of nutritional balance and scope. The danger is, of course, that these assumptions are based on the day's menu being a true representation of the habitual diet.

This particular case is a good example to explore food intake, in relation to socio-economic grouping; the case asks you to consider the likely nutritional implications of menus served on the *RMS Titanic* on 14 April 1912, one to first class passengers (served on B Deck) and one to third class passengers (served on F Deck).

Study questions

(1) Inspect the following menus and comment on the range and likely quality of foods served, in relation to the socio-economic grouping of the recipients. Remember to note these menus were served nearly 100 years ago, and it may be necessary to consider likely food availability a century ago.

(2) Imagine you were on board the ship. Make choices from each menu and compare and contrast the nutrient content they are likely to provide the consumer. You should eyeball the menus only. What conclusions can be drawn from these comparisons? You should focus on the likely balance of the intakes, assuming that menus represent typical foods eaten habitually.

Menu First Class, served on B Deck

14 April 1912
Last meals served on the ship

Breakfast
baked apples – fruit – steamed prunes
Quaker oats – boiled hominy – puffed rice
fresh herring – Finnan haddock – smoked salmon
grilled mutton – kidneys and bacon – grilled ham – grilled sausage
lamb callops – vegetable stew
fried, poached and boiled eggs – plain and tomato omelettes
sirloin steaks and mutton chops
mashed, sauté and jacket potatoes
cold meat and watercress
Vienna and Graham rolls
soda and sultana scones – corn bread – buckwheat cakes
blackcurrant conserve – Narbonne honey – Oxford marmalade

Lunch
consommé Fermier or Cock-a-Leekie
fillets of brill
chicken a la Maryland
corned beef, vegetables, dumplings

from the grill:
mutton chops
mashed, fried and jacket potatoes
custard pudding – apple meringue and pastry

from the buffet:
salmon mayonnaise – potted shrimps
Norwegian anchovies – soused herrings – smoked sardines

roast beef – spiced beef – veal and ham pie
Bologna sausage – brawn
galantine of chicken – corned ox tongue
lettuce – beetroot – tomatoes
Cheshire – Stilton – Camembert – Cheddar cheeses

Dinner
First course
canapés a l'admiral – oysters a la Russe
white Bordeaux or Burgundy

Second course
consommé Olga – cream of barley soup
Madeira or Sherry

Third course
poached salmon with mousseline sauce
dry Rhine wine or Moselle

Entrée course
filet mignon Lili – sauté of chicken Lyonnaise
vegetable marrow farcie
red Bordeaux

Fifth course
lamb with mint sauce
Calvados-glazed roast duckling with apple sauce
roast sirloin of beef Forrèstiere – chateau potatoes
minted pea timbales – creamed carrots – boiled rice – Parmentier and boiled new potatoes
red Burgundy or Beaujolais

Sixth course
Punch romaine (sorbet)

Seventh course
roasted squab on wilted cress
red Burgundy

Eighth course
cold asparagus salad with Champagne-saffron vinaigrette

Ninth course
pâté de foie gras
Sauterne or sweet Rhine wine

Tenth course
Waldorf pudding – peaches in Chartreuse jelly
chocolate painted éclairs with French vanilla cream – vanilla ice cream
Muscatel, Tokay and Sauterne wines

Eleventh course
assorted fresh fruits and cheeses
sweet dessert wines, Champagne and sparkling wines

After dinner
coffee, cigars with port or cordials

Menu Third Class, served on F Deck

10 April 1912

Breakfast
Quaker oats and milk
smoked herrings
beefsteak and onions
jacket potatoes
fresh bread and butter
Swedish bread
marmalade
tea – coffee

Lunch
brawn
cheese and pickles
fresh bread and butter
rhubarb jam
currant buns
tea

Dinner
rice soup
corned beef and cabbage
fresh or salt fish (as opportunity offers)
Kosher meat cooked for Jewish passengers as desired
boiled potatoes
cabin biscuits, fresh bread
peaches and rice

Case 34 Maria von Twigg

Anorexia nervosa

Study concepts: assessment of diet in an eating disordered client ■ the role of the dietitian ■ clinical outcomes in client group ■ likely prognosis

Study context: anorexia nervosa

Maria von Twigg is a 19-year-old international model who collapsed on the runway (catwalk) of a recent promotional fashion show. She was rushed to hospital with bradycardia, reduced pulse rate and hypotension. Tests later revealed mild thyroid dysfunction, anaemia and hypercholesterolaemia. She weighed 50 kg and is about 1.70 m, which is characteristic of the size zero shape (dress size 4, UK). She is irritable most of the time, pale, and works out in a local gymnasium about once or twice every day.

Maria was later admitted to a London clinic, a specialist facility for the treatment of anorexia nervosa.

Questions to consider

(1) Ms von Twigg is referred to see a dietitian as part of a programme designed to reduce risk of further exacerbation of symptoms associated with weight loss. What might be the dietary/nutritional strategy both in the short and longer term for this client?

(2) Explain the broader management plan or options available to stem weight loss or indeed increase weight in a client of this type.

(3) Discuss the possible stages in approach to assist the client through rehabilitation and discharge, to minimise risk of treatment relapse.

Study questions

(1) Discuss the extent to which you believe that a dietitian can assist a client such as Ms von Twigg.

(2) What particular skills might a dietitian need to be able to effect a good clinical outcome in a client such as this?

(3) Consider the clinical outcomes recommended for such a client. How many of these are associated with food and which may be managed most effectively by a dietitian?

(4) Comment on the peer-pressure that may result in the emergence of the size zero culture.

(5) Size zero is a term generated by the fashion industry. Classify this dress size 4 in terms of BMI (waist circumference 56 cm).

(6) Discuss the multi-disciplinary management of eating disorders and describe the individual roles of each member of the team.

Case 35 Alan Wanderlust

Colorectal cancer

Study concepts: therapeutic dietary issues ■ justification of nutritional management during pre-, peri- and post-operative periods in colorectal cancer

Study context: colorectal cancer ■ weight loss

Alan Wanderlust is a young veterinary surgeon (aged 38 years) who works alone in a rural practice in the Derbyshire Peak District. He has a recent history of abdominal pain and weight loss (8 kg in six months) which he has put down to 'drinking a little more then he should', paying 'absolutely no attention to his general diet' and stress. He eats when he can fit it in and lives predominantly on convenience foods. He lives alone in a small flat above the practice. His family history revealed that his father died of bowel problems. He is a keen walker and likes to walk in the Peaks.

The passage of black stools (melaena) and increasing epigastric pain prompted Alan to go to his general practitioner. Following referral to his nearest general hospital for tests, a colonoscopy revealed the presence of Dukes' B colorectal carcinoma. He will shortly undergo surgical resection of the tumour (in four weeks) together with adjuvant radiotherapy.

Questions to consider

(1) Mr Wanderlust is admitted two days before his surgery for blood work and further tests. Discuss the dietary intervention options available to him during this pre-operative period.
(2) Explain nutritional treatment goals that might be appropriate following surgery in the peri-operative and post-operative period.
(3) What might be the longer-term management options regarding Alan's diet that may be written up as part of discharge planning?

Study questions

(1) Describe Dukes' classification of bowel tumours. What does it tell you? Comment on its ability to inform treatment resources and identify prognosis.
(2) Discuss the methods available to predict clinical risk in a group of individuals susceptible to this condition.
(3) Explain the effects on appetite (and therefore voluntary and spontaneous oral intake) of radiotherapy.

Case 36 George and Dragon

Dementia, weight loss

Study concepts: therapeutic dietary issues ■ justification of nutritional management during assessment in hospital ■ managing nutritional support on a fluid restriction

Study context: dementia ■ weight loss

A 91-year-old man with mild dementia is admitted to hospital following a fall. His oral intake of food and drink is poor (about 600 kcal/d), and he tends to restrict his dietary intake to sweet foods, such as biscuits, and sweetened tea. He lives on his own, although a neighbour pops in regularly to take him for walks, do his shopping and take him for a game of dominoes at the *George and Dragon.*

His serum albumin concentration is low (25 g/l) and as a consequence he has developed oedema. He requires nutritional support but is also on fluid restriction of 1000 ml/d (failing renal function). He has lost 8 kg in weight over the past three months. His current weight is 45 kg (height 1.68 m).

Questions to consider

(1) Explain the likely cause of this fellow's poor nutritional status and recommend (with justification) short-term goals that will assist him to achieve his nutritional requirements.

(2) Calculate his major nutritional requirements and explain how these may be achieved by oral hospital diet.

(3) You elect to supplement his diet with sip feed(s). Consider how this will be implemented and discuss fully the factors that need to be taken into account.

(4) You discover that the sip feed(s) you have recommended and planned for the client remain on the patient's bedside locker or are accumulating in a ward refrigerator. What might be your plan of action?

(5) Explain the main elements of monitoring food and drink intake of a client such as this case.

Study questions

(1) A student nurse asks for an explanation of the connection between serum albumin and oedema. Outline the main points that may be made to her.

(2) In a case such as this, how can you increase the likelihood of the client continuing nutritional support at home?

(3) Supposing the client goes on to develop a pressure sore on one buttock, how may this affect nutritional requirements and why?

(4) Explain the purpose of assessing a patient's nutritional risk at baseline and at the various points in the treatment/care process.

Case 37 Mandy Morton

Ventilated patient, enteral feeding

Study concepts: calculation of nutritional requirements including stress factors ■ justification of selection of appropriate feeding regimen ■ monitoring methods and arrangements

Study context: enteral feeding ■ normal weight but stressed individual

Mandy Morton is an 18-year-old university student studying law. She plays in competitive hockey matches. Her mother was concerned about a recent episode of sickness and was shocked to hear that she had been taken into the high dependency unit of the local hospital with suspected meningitis.

Mandy is being ventilated and requires complete nutritional support. Her temperature is 39°C. Her height and weight have been recorded (1.60 m, 54 kg). As far as is known, the patient has a stable weight and has no history of weight loss.

Questions to consider

(1) Identify and discuss the nutritional care plan for this client, indicating clearly the short- and longer-term objectives.
(2) Calculate her major nutritional requirements and consider the feeding options that may be pursued in establishing enteral feeding.
(3) Design an appropriate regimen so that the client is able to achieve short-term nutritional goals.
(4) Suggest appropriate monitoring methods for this client, explaining clearly the objectives of each of the methods.

Study questions

(1) What might be considered as the chief clinical outcomes for normal weight patients receiving enteral feeding?
(2) Explain why an increase in core body temperature affects nutritional requirements and must be considered in both nursing and nutritional care.
(3) What considerations need to be thought about when selecting a suitable feeding regimen for clients fed enterally?

Case 38 Betty Meldrew

Breast cancer, weight loss

Study concepts: therapeutic dietary issues ■ justification of nutritional management during pre- and post-operative periods in cancer of the breast ■ dietary management and symptom resolution

Study context: breast cancer ■ weight loss

Betty Meldrew is a retired legal secretary and keeps herself busy at the local bowling club (where she often has her meals) and she has just become a local master bridge player at the Wellington Bridge Club. She was recently admitted to hospital for investigation and following tests has had a radical lumpectomy for cancer of the breast. She is now receiving a course of chemotherapy.

Betty's *appetite is poor*, she is *nauseated*, and she has noticed that she *cannot tolerate certain foods*, especially meat and fish. She has a *heightened sense of smell* and cannot bear the smell of cooked foods. She is *losing weight* (10 kg over the past two months).

Questions to consider

(1)   What might be the nutritional goals for Mrs Meldrew both in the short and longer term?
(2)   Assuming she is to be fed using oral hospital diet, and/or sip feeds, what might be the approaches taken to ensure that she receives an intake to meet her nutritional requirements?
(3)   Mrs Meldrew begins to reject the supplements provided and the oncology dietitian decides that a more aggressive approach might achieve requirements. She recommends a course of nocturnal nasogastric feeding to supplement oral diet, to provide an additional 1000 kcal/d. Calculate a possible feed to help the patient to meet her requirements.

Study questions

(1)   Outline the possible causes of the symptoms presented by Mrs Meldrew (these are italicised in the text).
(2)   Taking each symptom in turn, construct brief, but explicit dietary advice to help reduce these symptoms.
(3)   Consider the practical advice that may help this client as her discharge date approaches.

Case 39 Sheila Borrowman
Chronic pancreatitis, diabetes

Study concepts: therapeutic dietary intervention issues ■ justification of nutritional management during pre- and post-surgical intervention ■ management of weight loss ■ compliance with medical instructions and dietary adherence

Study context: chronic pancreatitis ■ weight loss and concomitant diabetes

Sheila Borrowman is a 61-year-old woman who was a practising dietitian until she started her family in her twenties. Her marriage became more and more difficult through the years until she eventually left her husband to live in a small but comfortable house in Prestatyn on the north Welsh coast.

She has a complex history but the most significant feature is that she underwent Whipple's procedure for chronic pancreatitis five years ago resulting in secondary diabetes. Though she has never fully admitted it, the doctors suspect that she has been misusing alcohol, coinciding with difficult periods in her life. She has become a bit of a recluse. Her diabetes is currently managed with insulin and she takes pancreatic enzymes, when she remembers.

The current history includes profound weight loss (10 kg over four months) and whilst this might relate to poor control of her diabetes and malabsorption, the physician suspects poor dietary intake. She protests that her diet is in good shape but the consultant wants more objective evidence that this is the case.

Questions to consider

(1) Discuss the approaches that may be taken and the selection of an appropriate dietary assessment that may be used in this case.
(2) The dietary assessment reveals an uneven pattern over the week and the client has good and bad days. Discuss how the client might be encouraged to take a more regular or consistent daily intake of food and why this might be an important longer-term goal.
(3) Briefly document a list of clinical priorities for Mrs Borrowman that may be important for her plan of care and follow-up.

Study questions

(1) Consider fully the evidence that implicates misuse of alcohol and poor eating patterns with incidence of chronic pancreatitis.
(2) Explain the likely symptomatology of patients prior to surgical resection and the methods of intervention used to manage these.
(3) Explore the indications for pancreatico-duodenectomy and comment on the likely prognosis of patients undergoing this aggressive procedure.

Case 40 Miss Taylor

Cancer of lung, cachexia

Study concepts: therapeutic dietary priorities ■ justification of nutritional management during acute care ■ discharge planning and follow-up arrangements

Study context: cancer of the lung ■ weight loss and cachexia

Miss Taylor is a retired company director's personal assistant and has recently celebrated her 75th birthday. She has kept reasonably well until her recent illness, when she was admitted to hospital with difficulty in breathing and a persistent and distressing cough. She is of average height and her admitting weight was 43.5 kg.

Miss Taylor is lucid and has an excellent memory. She has been a heavy smoker all her life and latterly she has been living on cigarettes and cups of tea. She lives on her own and has lost interest in herself, but keeps herself busy with her favourite pastimes of crochet and tatting.

A diagnosis of emphysema is made secondary to cancer of the lung and she is scheduled to have a resection performed in the next week or so. She is surprisingly interested in the hospital diet.

Questions to consider

(1)   Explain the dietary priorities for Miss Taylor, justifying fully the nature of dietary intervention that may appear in a care plan.
(2)   State and calculate the principal nutritional requirements for the patient and document a case note entry based on the history outlining fully how the patient may meet nutritional requirements by appropriate and practical dietary intervention.
(3)   Suggest how the patient may be followed up and how compliance with a new diet may be monitored.

Study questions

(1)   Explore the pathology of emphysema and the implications this may have for clinical care.
(2)   Explain and fully discuss the nature and development of cancer cachexia and how this may be ameliorated by aggressive dietary intervention.
(3)   How can interest in food be maintained in a client such as Miss Taylor as she returns to her own home?

Case 41 Mary Glover

Coeliac disease, lymphoma

Study concepts: therapeutic dietary issues ■ justification of nutritional management during peri-operative period ■ longer-term care ■ patients lost to follow-up

Study context: lymphoma and coeliac disease ■ management of a post-surgical patient

Mary Glover is a 46-year-old housewife who helps with Radio Lollipop, a local children's hospital radio station. She has had ongoing abdominal discomfort stretching back into her young adulthood, and this was diagnosed as irritable bowel disease when at that time she had a very demanding job as a prison officer in a young person's unit. Recently, she has begun to feel rather unwell and presented to her GP with nausea, much more diarrhoea than usual and occasional rectal bleeding. She reports the presence of bone pain and weight loss. She is referred to the gastroenterology unit for investigation.

After an upper and lower bowel series of tests, it is discovered that Mrs Glover has a fairly aggressive bowel lymphoma secondary to a missed diagnosis of coeliac disease. This is complicated by the presence of osteoporosis. The surgeon elects to resect the tumour. The procedure is uneventful and the patient is expected to make a full recovery.

Questions to consider

(1) Assuming the patient is admitted as a clinical priority and the patient is referred for dietary review following surgery, sketch out the short- and longer-term nutritional goals for Mrs Glover.

(2) Comment fully on feeding the post-surgical patient during the peri-operative phase, and indicate when this patient might benefit from initial exposure to the dietitian.

(3) Discuss the nature and extent of follow-up that may be appropriate, and explain why.

(4) Should the patient be lost to follow-up, explain the action(s) that might be considered appropriate for the dietitian, to assist in achievement of clinical outcomes.

Study questions

(1) Explain the epidemiology of a diagnosis of irritable bowel syndrome induced by stress.

(2) Consider the development of osteoporosis in a case such as this and explain how this can be managed medically, nutritionally and through lifestyle changes.

(3) Explain the phenomenon of clients who are 'lost to follow-up' and consider methods that may be employed as alternatives to clinic attendance.

Case 42 Pamela Nightingale

Chronic fatigue syndrome

Study concepts: therapeutic and alternative dietary issues ■ justification of diet and lifestyle management ■ evidence-based versus alternative therapy interventions

Study context: chronic fatigue syndrome ■ management of tiredness

Pamela Nightingale is a 43-year-old full-time nurse who works in a long-stay care home for older persons. She also 'dabbles in homoeopathy' and advertises her services in shops and in the local weekly newspaper. She describes herself as an informed pavement therapist. She is generally well despite coping with fibromyalgia but has recently suffered from a myalgic encephalomyopathy-type virus infection which has resulted in a flare up of her arthritis. She reports tiredness and a post-prandial energy slump as significant features. Her sleep pattern is disturbed (apnoea) and is therefore of poor quality. She does no exercise and goes everywhere by car.

Pamela is 5 ft 0 in in height and her weight is approximately 80 kg. Over the years she has suspected various adverse reactions to food but only lactose intolerance has been clinically diagnosed. She has become an enthusiastic vegetarian and seeks advice about how she might be able to resolve constant tiredness through dietary means.

Questions to consider

(1) Based on the available scientific evidence, justify the possible diet and lifestyle approaches that may be indicated for Mrs Nightingale.
(2) Explain the connection between these approaches and the potential for these to resolve, at least in part, some of the symptoms experienced by the client.

Study questions

(1) Compare and contrast the diagnoses of chronic fatigue syndrome and lactose intolerance in the context of scientific credibility.
(2) Comment on the extent to which homoeopathy might assist in the care of clients with chronic fatigue, again through the eyes of the scientific community.
(3) Explain the position of the wider application of homoeopathy to assist in health care delivery and the extent to which health care practitioners need to embrace the role of alternative medicine.

Case 43 Jenny Friel

Crohn's disease

Study concepts: dietary issues to achieve weight maintenance ■ nutritional management with and without corticosteroid use ■ chronic disease management and eating behaviours

Study context: Crohn's disease ■ weight maintenance

Jenny Friel is a 20-year-old geography student at Aberdeen University who is currently on a placement in Dubai on a mapping assignment. A diagnosis of terminal ileal and caecal Crohn's disease was made two years previously. She has been largely intolerant of various medications and is currently on no long-term prophylaxis, although she has been on high-dose maintenance corticosteroids during the early stages of her diagnosis. She has tried eliminating wheat-containing foods and is extremely intolerant of fatty foods. She has been experiencing weight loss recently, and her current BMI is 27 kg/m². The consultant is keen to prevent further weight loss. The patient announces that she is to be married in a few months.

Ms Friel reacted quite badly to establishment of corticosteroids at the age of 13 years, having heard that they result in weight gain. Although compliant with these drugs, she aggressively pursued any means available to counter or resist weight gain (excessive exercising and considerable dietary restraint). Thus, she embarked upon a self-imposed regimen of a fat-free diet, with daily visits to the gym.

Questions to consider

(1) Discuss the approaches that may be made to determine current dietary patterns and intake.
(2) Consider the significant dietary components that may be of interest to investigate and explain how this information may guide therapeutic intervention. What are the dietary priorities for this client?
(3) Explain the nature of possible food intolerances and how these can be managed to effect weight maintenance.

Study questions

(1) Explain the role and function of the use of corticosteroids in the management of Crohn's disease.
(2) Consider the young female client who may resist any clinical intervention that may result in weight gain. How can this tension be diffused without the very aggressive attempts shown by this client to moderate the effects of medical intervention?
(3) Anorexia may be a consequence of longer-term patients with Crohn's disease and is associated with poor clinical outcome. Explain this phenomenon and how it might be avoided.

Case 44 Alan Lehman

Type 1 diabetes

Study concepts: therapeutic dietary issues ■ prioritisation of dietary improvements justification ■ evidence-based lifestyle recommendations ■ dietary adherence issues

Study context: longstanding diabetes ■ diet and lifestyle change

Alan Lehman (44 years old) is a part-time manager of a local, small, professional football team and considers himself as one of the boys and claims to
be fit. He was recently awarded the title of league 'Manager of the year'.
Although his general health is good, he is annoyed that his weight is beginning to creep up (currently 103.9 kg with a waist circumference of 98 cm).

Alan has had diabetes for some 20 years and is currently taking Novo-
Rapid (18 units) before each meal and 18 units of Lantus at night. His HbA$_{1c}$
level is 8.1% and is down from previous values. He does not experience
hypoglycaemia.

Alan takes simvastatin (20 mg), which is working well, and his total cholesterol is 3.74 mmol/l with an HDL cholesterol level of 1.53 mmol/l. Liver and
renal function is within normal limits. His blood pressure is excellent at
126/60 mmHg. He also takes 75 mg aspirin and 20 mg lisinopril daily. He is
shortly to have a retinal screen and has been referred for dietary assessment
and intervention.

Questions to consider

(1) Consider the above information that has been extracted from the
patient's case notes. Comment fully on the clinical information presented, with reference to each parameter and linking this with any
associated health risk(s).
(2) Critically analyse the information and prioritise the dietary and lifestyle
modifications that may feature as part of a review appointment.
(3) Compare and contrast the approach that may be taken during the therapeutic interview as determined by whether the client is motivated or
unmotivated to improve his health by diet and lifestyle intervention.

Study questions

(1) Consider the government's recommendations or guidelines concerned
with physical activity and alcohol consumption. How can the general
public be persuaded to follow these guidelines?
(2) Explore the evidence linking hypertension with salt (sodium) intake. Turn
this information into practical advice in the form of a leaflet, remember-
ing to include a section justifying the level of restriction. The information
should be motivational, to assist change in dietary behaviour.

Case 45 Mark

Attention deficit hyperactivity disorder

Study concepts: re-alignment of dietary pattern to improve behaviour ■ exploration of
evidence implicating dietary improvement with behavioural management

Study context: diet in ADHD ■ growth failure ■ parental responsibility

Mark is an 11-year-old boy who has ADHD. He is described by his mother as being angelic and a cherub from the outside, but on the inside he is precocious and high spirited! His behaviour has improved with a combination of methylphenidate (Ritalin) and a programme of cognitive behavioural therapy delivered by the clinical psychologist. He is of small stature and is being reviewed by a physician at the Sick Children's Hospital for FTT.

His mother is very concerned about his eating habits as they continue to cause havoc at meal times. In addition, there is evidence that he is being bullied at school because he is so small in relation to his peers. His weight struggles to achieve the lower end of the 25–50th centile. He has been extensively investigated for hormonal causes of growth failure but no significant pathology has been found. His mother is of small build but the biological father (he is living with his mother and step-father) is tall (185 cm). Mark and his mother attend an outpatient clinic following referral by the FTT team.

Questions to consider

(1) Discuss the approach you might take to inspect Mark's eating habits more fully.
(2) Prioritise the information you may want to explore to help arrive at a judgement about whether there may be a link between his diet and growth failure.
(3) You discover that Mark is a picky eater; he eats about half the food that is offered to him and is often caught pilfering food from cupboards and biscuit tins between meals. His breakfast and school lunch and snacks are unsupervised. What advice might you give the mother and perhaps school personnel?
(4) You also find out that Mark's meals consist of quickly prepared foods, such as fried sausages, fish fingers, cakes and pastries and he consumes little in the way of fruit and vegetables. Advocate and justify a new diet for Mark in an attempt to reduce the likelihood of his diet impacting on either growth failure, ADHD and/or general health.

Study question

(1) Propose a strategy for involving the school in assisting with improving dietary intake and pattern.

Case 46 Mary Montgomery and Mary Hamilton

Oral pathology, nutritional issues

Study concepts: ethical issues surrounding feeding the nutritionally compromised elderly ■ justification of nutritional goal setting in complicated and uncomplicated oral/oesophageal lesions ■ issues related to monitoring of dietary intake

Study context: oral pathology and related nutritional issues

Mary Montgomery is an 85-year-old woman residing in a care home situated in a suburb of Cardiff. She has long-standing, but well-controlled Parkinson's disease and has recently developed reflux oesophagitis. She is not confined to bed, and is losing weight. Her appetite is good, but her memory is not, hence many of the sip feeds prescribed for her remain unfinished or unopened on her locker. She weighs 65 kg.

Mary Hamilton is a frail elderly woman (aged 84 years, weight 43.5 kg) who was admitted to a general medical ward following a fall in the snow. She sustained a scaphoid fracture of her right hand together with multiple fractures of her left hip. Her appetite has been poor for some months and it is discovered she has cancer of the tongue. Radical surgical resection of the tumour is performed and high-dose radiotherapy commenced.

Questions to consider

(1) Compare and contrast the two patients with regard to their diagnosis and physical condition, and discuss the implications that help inform short-term nutritional goals.
(2) Justify the preferred method of feeding both clients and comment fully on the likelihood of meeting short-term goals mentioned in Question (1).
(3) Comment fully on the issues related to monitoring dietary intake presented by each of the patients.
(4) Discuss any ethical issues presented by each of the cases, looking particularly at the weight of evidence governing feeding, prognosis and quality of life.

Study questions

(1) Consider the pathologies and medical management associated with both parkinsonism and cancer of the tongue and make a few notes on the impact of the symptoms on nutritional management.
(2) How might the nutritional status and assessment of nutritional risk be estimated in both patients? Which methods are more valid or reliable, which are more practical and least invasive, in determining nutritional status or nutritional risk?

Case 47 Sara Bloomfield

Chronic obstructive airways disease

Study concepts: dietary adherence to increased energy requirements with diet disinterest ■ maintaining interest in diet in light of social isolation ■ dietary tension in household

Study context: chronic obstructive airways disease ■ increased energy requirements

Sara Bloomfield is a 72-year-old woman who is currently undergoing pulmonary rehabilitation with the physiotherapist as part of treatment for COPD. She had a forced expiratory volume of 0.6 litres (28%) some weeks ago and this has improved by about 250 ml to 0.9 litres (42%) following introduction of a beta-2 agonist. Her oxygen saturation is satisfactory (94% on air). She is now prescribed tiotropium (18 mg/d) and Salamol Easi-Breathe (salbutamol) (six hourly or on an as required basis).

Mrs Bloomfield has a persistent, hacking cough and frequent infections treated with antibiotics. Her current weight is causing concern (BMI 14.8 kg/m^2) and she is referred to the dietitian. During the consultation it is discovered that there is tension in the household over meals and eating. Mrs Bloomfield's husband is permanently on a diet in order to lose weight (he has rheumatoid arthritis), and she refers to him as Jack Spratt ('could eat no fat . . .'). She eats alone ('. . . his wife could eat no lean') and confines her eating to meal times only. She has no real interest in food, but forces herself to sit down to have a meal. Breakfast consists of an egg on toast, lunch is usually soup and a roll and her evening meal is always a two-course meal, consisting of meat or fish with vegetables, followed by a dessert. She eats traditional food.

Questions to consider

(1) Explain the connection between the physical features of the condition and nutritional requirements.
(2) Discuss the short- and longer-term nutritional goals for Mrs Bloomfield and consider fully how the patient may be able to incorporate these practically into her regular diet.

Study questions

(1) Consider the drugs prescribed for this patient and indicate the likely impact of these on management of the condition.
(2) Explain what might be the effect of antibiotic use on nutritional status.

Case 48 Jonny Morgan

Thinness, faulty diet and health risk

Study concepts: alignment of diet with eating frequency recommendations ■ assessment of health risk of dietary pattern and lifestyle ■ link between sodium intake and hypertension

Study context: thinness ■ health risk

Jonny Morgan works on a fruit and vegetable stall in a local indoor market. He works 12-hr shifts which involves not only selling but replenishing stock from packing crates. He is a very outgoing fellow, but viewed by his work-mates as being too thin. He is otherwise healthy but has a BMI of 14.5 kg/m² and is now a little concerned about his body image. He is 19 years of age and is constantly being 'ribbed' about his shape. He has always been thin and comes from a family where his mother and father are both thin. He smokes 40 cigarettes/d.

After a 6 am to 6 pm shift, Jonny can be found most evenings in his local pub, staying until about 10 pm. This is usually followed by a supper from the local deep fry shop (battered fish or deep fried pizza, with chips) on the way home. He starts his day with a large fry-up of bacon and egg, sausages and fried bread. He has little to eat throughout the day, except for mugs of strong, sweetened, milky coffee.

Jonny approaches his GP about his weight and he is referred on to the dietitian.

Questions to consider

(1) Discuss the possible approaches that may be taken in trying to realign his diet with a more appropriate eating pattern and food selection.
(2) Assess the possible risk to longer-term health if the current dietary intake and pattern was to continue.
(3) Consider the lifestyle changes that may benefit Jonny's general health and explain why these might assist reducing his cardiovascular health risk.
(4) What particular approaches may be taken to assess dietary intake of salt and how would intake determine overall health risk?

Study questions

(1) Explain the possible association that may exist between eating frequency and health.
(2) If eating practices for this client fail to change, and he goes on to develop essential hypertension, explain the evidence that implicates sodium intake and attempt to quantify the possible benefits from appropriate dietary intervention.

Case 49 Patrick Foley

Burn injury

Study concepts: nutrition support in burn injury ■ meeting increased nutritional requirements during appetite failure ■ provision of adequate oral diet ■ metabolic response to trauma

Study context: burn injury ■ nutritional support

Patrick Foley is a 24-year-old car dealer who works 'on the floor' of a large sports car dealership. He keeps himself physically fit (85 kg, 170 cm) and regularly plays amateur ice hockey for a local team. He was involved in a house fire recently and was extensively burned, with injury predominantly to his upper body (arms, chest and back) and legs (back and front). He was taken to the local accident and emergency unit where his burns were assessed as both partial and full-thickness over 30% of his body surface. He was then taken to the regional burns unit for re-assessment and ongoing treatment.

Mr Foley was treated initially for shock and pain relief. A central venous line was inserted and fluid replacement therapy begun. Fluid and electrolyte status were monitored; his blood pressure duly improved. He was nil-by-mouth and prophylactic antibiotics were administered. The wounds were debrided and dressed. On day 3 post-burn, his urine output improved dramatically, as diuresis was established. Oral diet was commenced. A long rehabilitation period is predicted (skin grafting). He remains chirpy, despite a poor appetite. You review him on day 4 and assess his oral diet to contain about 3.3 MJ (800 kcal).

Questions to consider

(1) Explain what might be Mr Foley's short-term nutritional goals following acute thermal injury.
(2) Using the clinical information and physical data that you are given, explain the factors that may be taken into account to meet his increased nutritional requirements.
(3) Estimate a daily dietary prescription in terms of protein, energy and fluid to meet his nutritional requirements.
(4) Give an account of practical considerations in providing suitable nutrition for Mr Foley.

Study questions

(1) Explain how the extent and depth of burn injury is calculated and how this is interpreted to provide a nutritional prescription.
(2) Account for the possible development of renal impairment in a case such as this.

Case 50 Doris Blessing

Type 2 diabetes, pressure sore

Study concepts: dietary adherence during wound crisis ■ care home priorities ■ management of poor nutritional status in a diabetic client ■ ongoing assessment and evaluation

Study context: type 2 diabetes ■ malnutrition ■ glycaemic control and wound healing

Doris Blessing is an 80-year-old spinster and a rather colourful character. She was born just before World War II into a warm and loving family and has had a very successful career as a travel correspondent and writer of a regular column in a national newspaper. She is rather deaf and until recently has been involved with activities where she sign-writes for other deaf people.

She developed type 2 diabetes in her sixties, which has been managed without the use of oral hypoglycaemic agents. Her glycaemic control and general health has been exemplary over the years despite two periods of hospitalisation for a flare-up of her arthritis (1995) and an elective cholecystectomy (1999). She is of average build and within the normal range of BMI. She has become more of a recluse in the past five years or so and 'keeps herself to herself' in a neat red-brick terraced house. She has become increasingly debilitated with arthritis and is unable to walk for any length of time. She has also become increasingly forgetful.

Doris was admitted to hospital for assessment following a visit by a district nurse to review her diabetes. She is anaemic, her blood albumin concentration is low (25 g/l) and she has lost weight recently (8 kg in six months). Her fasting blood glucose level was 12 mmol/l. She has a pressure sore over her sacrum and is nursed on a water bed, turned hourly, and resting on sheepskins.

Questions to consider

(1) Explain what might be the nutritional care plan for Doris and indicate, with justification, the short and longer term's goals for her.
(2) What might be her requirements for protein and energy on initial assessment and explain how these will be achieved.
(3) After two weeks in hospital, the decision is made to look for a place in a care home where she can remain relatively independent. What guidance for the carers might be considered appropriate in terms of nutrition?

Study questions

(1) Explain the link between the presence of a pressure sore and worsening glycaemic control.
(2) Consider the position of the care home. What quality assurance mechanism(s) preside(s) over a residential home to deliver optimum nutritional care?

Case 51 Rupert St. John Stevens

Alcoholic liver disease

Study concepts: nutritional requirements ■ liver function and nutritional status ■ monitoring in a chronic condition ■ interpretation of clinical data ■ appropriate approaches in alcohol clients

Study context: alcoholic cirrhosis ■ nutritional status ■ dry weight

Rupert St. John Stevens is an antique dealer who owns his own shop (All that glitters) in an exclusive part of town. He is 56 years old and is divorced. His two married sons live nearby and have become increasingly concerned about his disinterest in food, associated weight loss and mild confusion. He is nauseated and complains of upper quadrant discomfort, which he puts down to a touch of heartburn. He has a tender abdomen which is later discovered to be hepatomegaly. He weighs 73.0 kg and has lost 8 kg in six months. It is estimated that he consumes about five to six units of alcohol every day, and is carrying about 4 litres fluid as abdominal ascites. He is assessed in hospital and the blood work reveals the following clinical chemistry:

Serum/plasma constituent	Result	Reference range
Albumin (g/l)	29	35–45
Bilirubin (µmol/l)	180	2–17
Glucose (mmol/l)	4.6	3.0–5.0
Haemoglobin (g/dl)	12.0	13.5–17.5 (male)
Potassium (mmol/l)	2.8	3.5–5.0
Prothrombin time (seconds)	35	12–15
Sodium (mmol/l)	135	135–150
Total protein (g/l)	58	60–80
ALP activity (u/l)	200	40–125
ALT activity (u/l)	50	10–40
AST activity (u/l)	55	10–34
GGT activity (u/l)	150	10–35

Questions to consider

(1) Explain the clinical information provided by the blood work. Summarise the significance of this in relation to his diagnosis (alcoholic liver disease).

(2) Draw up a nutritional care plan for the client in terms of short- and longer-term goals.

(3) Assess his nutrient requirements and discuss practical approaches to meet these using the hospital diet as the basis of nutritional care.

(4) Prioritise the practical advice that may be given to the client as part of discharge planning, to maintain a good state of nutrition.

(5) Discuss the monitoring arrangements that may be put into place to ensure that further damage to the liver is avoided.

Case 52 Mrs Morningside

Chronic peptic ulceration

Study concepts: short- and longer-term issues related to dyspepsia ■ iron deficiency anaemia ■ vitamin B$_{12}$ deficiency ■ weight loss ■ partial gastrectomy and potential dietary restrictions

Study context: dyspepsia ■ peptic ulcer disease ■ anaemia

Kathy Morningside is a 55-year-old woman who has had spells of gastrointestinal problems over the years (dyspepsia), but a formal diagnosis has never been conclusive. During the past four months, she has had a history of vomiting after some meals and she has lost about 5 kg over this time.

Mrs Morningside, together with an old school chum, went to London for a weekend theatre break to see *Les Miserables*. On the Friday evening, she began to feel unwell, but put it down to her fear of flying. They went to the theatre on the Saturday evening and followed this with a light opera supper at a nearby restaurant. Mrs Morningside suffered a haematemesis and was rushed to hospital with massive bleeding. Her condition settled and following overnight rehydration, she returned to her home in Newcastle where she was examined by a gastrointestinal consultant.

The consultant noted that Mrs Morningside was pale and tachycardic. Her blood pressure was 130/90 mmHg. Rectal examination revealed frank melaena. He attributed the bleed to chronic peptic ulceration, probably as a consequence of long-term use of non-specific anti-inflammatory drugs. He considers her to be at high risk of re-bleeding and may contemplate partial gastrectomy when her nutritional intake has improved.

The consultant refers Mrs Morningside to the dietitian as he is concerned about her overall nutritional status. She is currently anaemic (frank iron and possibly megaloblastic/pernicious anaemia).

Questions to consider

(1) Explain the approaches that may be taken to assess this patient's nutritional and dietary status.

(2) Consider the dietary assessment more carefully. What may be the principal focus of the interview with the client? What advance preparation might assist you in the conduct of the assessment interview?

(3) Advocate the nutritional goals for this client to achieve better nutritional status.

(4) Explain the practical measures that may assist the client in achieving these goals.

(5) If the patient goes on to have a partial gastrectomy as a prophylactic measure to reduce risk of bleeding, what particular nutritional issues might this raise in the longer term?

(6) Explain how the nutritional goals in Question (3) would now be influenced following surgery (Question (5)) and discuss the monitoring that might assist the dietitian in judging whether these goals are being met.

Study questions

(1) Discuss the incidence of peptic ulcer disease, considering fully how the medical and nutritional management has changed with time to present clinical guidelines.

(2) Explain the role of the stomach in maintaining optimum iron status and consider also its role in preventing pernicious anaemia.

(3) Explain fully the concept of dumping syndrome and indicate how it may be managed by dietary means.

(4) Draw up a possible (and brief) diet plan for a client with dumping.

Case 53 Mandy Goodenough

Gestational diabetes

Study concepts: pattern of growth in pregnancy ■ management of poor glycaemic control ■ weight management in pregnancy ■ the African Caribbean diet

Study context: gestational diabetes ■ glycaemic control and weight gain

Mandy Goodenough is of African Caribbean origin and a full-time hairdresser and beautician in a local beauty salon. She is 26 years of age and is a primipara at 25 weeks' gestation and beginning to feel tired. She visits her GP and after routine tests she is diagnosed with anaemia and gestational diabetes. She is also constipated. She lives with her partner in a small flat above the salon, but due to his job he is away a lot. Her dietary history reveals an intake of about 3000 kcal/d and she consumes a largely European diet, but traditional dietary items are consumed when available (such as sugary biscuits and cakes, plantain and rice). She maintains a traditional dietary pattern of two meals each day (omitting lunch) and her large evening meal is usually a stew, containing coconut milk or peanuts. She adores vegetables.

Mandy knows she was carrying excess weight at the outset of pregnancy and is keen not to put on too much as she has heard that this may produce a big baby.

Her weight history is as follows:

Weight history	Weight (kg)
Usual preconception weight (self-reported)	80.2
Weight at 6 weeks (GP)	83.2
Weight at 14 weeks (booking clinic and scan)	87.4
Weight at 20 weeks (self-reported)	89.6
Weight at 25 weeks (GP)	94.0

Questions to consider

(1) Inspect the weight history data and give a commentary on the pattern of weight to date, comparing this with ideal weight patterning.
(2) Discuss the nutritional goals throughout the remaining pregnancy and formulate an action plan for the client.
(3) How might Mandy's constipation be managed?
(4) Had Mandy been seen at a pre-conceptual clinic, what nutritional and lifestyle guidance might have been given to her and why?

Study questions

(1) Explain the connection between iron medication and development of constipation.
(2) What are the chief characteristics of the traditional African Caribbean diet and explain any potential influences on health risk/benefits that may be associated with this type of diet.
(3) Write an account of optimal weight gain during pregnancy and why this may be important.

Case 54 Mrs Jessie Banks
Renal disease, type 2 diabetes

Study concepts: dietary intervention ■ management of symptomatology ■ conservative management ■ discharge planning and follow-up arrangements

Study context: chronic renal failure ■ pre-dialysis ■ type 2 diabetes

Mrs Jessie Banks is a 64-year-old woman who leads a busy life – she has one passion in life – she shows her prize-winning Pomeranians. She has become increasingly tired over the past few months. Her friends have remarked that she is getting thinner and that she is generally out of sorts. She has noticed that she is passing more urine than usual, and has to get up in the middle of the night. She decided to have a check up by her GP.

The GP noted that Mrs Banks was pale and her blood pressure was 180/115. Her weight at consultation was 60.1 kg (height 1.60 m). Urinalysis revealed protein and glucose. Her blood work was as follows:

Serum/plasma constituent	Result	Reference range
Alkaline phosphatase activity (u/l)	226	40–125
Calcium (mmol/l)	1.88	2.25–2.65
Creatinine (µmol/l)	635	40–130
Glucose (mmol/l)	6.2	3.0–5.0
Haemoglobin (g/dl)	9.2	11.5–15.5 (female)
Phosphate (mmol/l)	2.38	0.8–1.4
Potassium (mmol/l)	5.4	3.5–5.0
Sodium (mmol/l)	129	135–150
Total carbon dioxide (mmol/l)	17	24–30
Urea (mmol/l)	38.2	3.3–6.7

Mrs Banks is referred to the medical renal unit for more extensive tests and is later diagnosed with chronic renal failure and type 2 diabetes. The initial plan is conservative management.

Questions to consider

(1) The patient is seen shortly after she is admitted to the renal unit. Outline appropriate short- and longer-term goals for Mrs Banks, justifying your decisions; devise a nutritional prescription and eating plan for her.

(2) You advise Mrs Banks how to select an appropriate range of foods from the hospital menu. Using the menu given below (Figure 3), make appropriate choices for her. (It may be useful to first copy the menu, and enter or write on the menu.) Provide a commentary on why you have made selections; where foods are inappropriate, write onto the menu card additional menu item(s) that may be provided by a main kitchen in order to meet her dietary requirements.

(3) Assuming she leaves hospital, describe a possible discharge plan for Mrs Banks, indicating clearly discharge and follow-up arrangements.

(4) She is reviewed in 12 months time and whilst her renal function is still viable, she has lost 5 kg from baseline. What dietary advice reinforcement may be necessary, and why?

Menu for Queen Victoria Hospital

Please circle numbers, portion sizes, indicating your choice

Cases

Ward: Name:		Room No:		Ward: Name:		Room No:		Ward: Name:		Room No:	
	BREAKFAST				LUNCH				DINNER		
portion	small	medium	large	portion	small	medium	large	portion	small	medium	large
01	fruit juice			01	Scotch broth			01	white sandwich		
02	Weetabix			02	mackerel pâté			02	wholemeal sandwich		
03	porridge			03				03	egg mayonnaise		
04	milk			04				04	tongue		
05				05	Cumberland pie			05	tomato		
06	poached egg			06	haggis			06	Grosvenor pie		
07	grilled bacon			07	cheese salad			07			
08				08				08	butter		
09	bread – white			09				09	margarine		
10	bread – wholemeal			10	mashed potato			10			
11	toast – white			11	chipped potato			11	salad bowl		
12	croissant			12	pureed peppered swede			12	Mediterranean dressing		
13				13				13	fresh fruit		
14				14	peas			14	raspberry Pavlova		
15	butter			15				15	bread – white		
16	margarine			16	caramel cream			16	bread granary		
17				17	vanilla ice cream			17	tea bread		
18	jam			18	sticky toffee pudding			18	butter		
19	marmalade			19	fresh fruit			19	margarine		
20	tea			20	tea			20	tea		
21	coffee			21	coffee			21	coffee		
22	milk			22	milk			22	milk		
23	sugar			23	sugar			23	sugar		

Figure 3 Sample hospital menu.

Study questions

(1) Study the clinical information given in the story, and explain the connection between pathology and symptoms.
(2) Examine the results of the blood work and explain why the clinical chemistry is consistent with the diagnosis of chronic renal failure.
(3) Consider the drugs that may assist in her medical care and clinical control and explain why each one may enhance her quality of life.

Case 55 Toby Harris

Fractured mandible

Study concepts: estimation of nutritional requirements in a well-nourished patient with acute injury ■ planning fluid diet using hospital diet ■ monitoring an ambulatory patient in hospital and as part of discharge planning

Study context: liquid nutrition during acute trauma

Toby Harris is an apprentice painter and decorator (aged 23 years). He attends a local college (day release) and is nearing completion of his apprenticeship. He is 6 ft 3 in and attends a gym three times a week. He is of slim build but at the upper end of the normal range of BMI, probably due to a high proportion of muscle. He is 'football daft' and is described by his friends as a bit of a hothead.

Following the final whistle at a local derby football match, Toby gets involved in a fight and is admitted to the accident and emergency department of the nearby general hospital. He has a compound fracture of mandible and pugilist fracture of his right hand. He is admitted to an orthopaedic ward for surgical repair of his mandible and review of his hand injury. He has intermaxillary fixation with wires to immobilise his jaw and these will remain *in situ* for a period of five to six weeks. He can accommodate a wide-bore flexi-straw. Nursing staff order a liquid diet.

Questions to consider

(1) Comment on Mr Harris's likely nutritional status at baseline, i.e. before the fight.
(2) Explain his nutritional goals and discuss the main objectives of care in the immediate six weeks' post-surgical period.
(3) Indicate his nutritional priorities and calculate his nutritional requirements.

(4)   Devise and plan a suitable intake to meet his nutritional requirements using a combination of liquids from the hospital diet and sip feeds.

(5)   Explain the approaches that may be taken to, firstly, establish the regimen and, secondly, maintain the intake during the period of hospitalisation.

(6)   Explain the advice that may be given as part of discharge planning.

Study questions

(1)   Discuss possible monitoring strategies that may be implemented as part of ward routine.

(2)   What particular difficulties may be experienced by a patient such as Mr Harris and explain how these may be overcome.

(3)   Explain the role of nutrition in bone health and healing.

Case 56 John Thomson

Motor neurone disease

Study concepts: estimation of nutritional requirements in progressive dysphagia ■ assisting nutritional intake in dysphagia ■ multi-disciplinary team care

Study context: progressive dysphagia ■ motor neurone disease

John Thomson is a devoted football fan of Leeds United, and indeed used to manage the youth team. He has a whole room in his house devoted to 'his teams' memorabilia. He is 62 years of age and has begun to notice stiffness in his fingers and a slight clumsiness in his walking but puts this down to rheumatism and getting older. His GP refers him to a neurologist who diagnoses early stage motor neurone disease. Mr Thomson is constipated and his mobility is impaired as a result of foot drop but his dietary intake remains relatively unchanged. His BMI is $24\,kg/m^2$ (73.2 kg) and his dietary intake causes no concern.

Mr Thomson's condition worsens and six months later his weight has fallen to 65 kg. He has some difficulty holding knives and forks and he has difficulty swallowing. He is seen by the occupational therapist who advises him on use of specialist cutlery. His condition further deteriorates and one year later, muscle atrophy affects his tongue and pharynx, as well as lower limbs. Though his cognitive function is relatively intact, he is unable to communicate orally and resorts to using a spelling board. He has become progressively dysphagic to most solid foods and to some liquids, and the SLT gives him safe swallow advice. His BMI is now $17.8\,kg/m^2$.

Questions to consider

At the six-month stage following diagnosis Mr Thomson's estimated oral intake is about 1000 kcal/d. He is dysphagic to bread, but is surprisingly able to tolerate meat and fish, biscuits and cereals. He is enthusiastic about milk, yoghurt, puddings and most drinks (hot and cold).

(1) Indicate the principal nutrients that are important in the nutritional care of Mr Thomson, and why.
(2) Assess his nutritional requirements and discuss the practical advice that is necessary to achieve these nutritional goals using a combination of regular diet, fluids and/or sip feeds.
(3) Discuss the possible monitoring methods that may assist in determining whether his nutritional requirements are being met.

At the 18-month stage following diagnosis, Mr Thomson is hospitalised and nutritional screening classifies him 'at risk' of malnutrition. His oral intake is assessed to be about 500 kcal/d and the decision made to feed him using gastrostomy.

(4) Re-assess his nutritional requirements and devise an appropriate feeding strategy. Explain how the strategy will deliver suitable nutrition.
(5) Consider the monitoring arrangements necessary and indicate how frequently these will be required and why.

Study questions

(1) Explain the development of signs and symptoms in motor neurone disease and indicate how members of the MDT may be involved in care of clients with this condition.
(2) Consider carefully how you might communicate with this patient as his condition progresses and explain the level of dialogue that you think might be helpful.

Case 57 Daisy Marsden
Alcoholic liver disease

Study concepts: interpretation of clinical information ■ therapeutic dietary issues ■ relationship between clinical chemistry and stage of disease ■ cholesterol-lowering strategies ■ strategies to reduce hypertension risk

Study context: alcoholic liver disease

Daisy Marsden owns her own florist's shop on the high street (Awesome Blossoms) and celebrated her 48th birthday last year. It had been a difficult year for her, following the sudden death of her partner of 30 years.

Review of her case notes reveals that she has had progressive worsening of liver function tests, although she only complains of fatigue, which she thinks is due to over-working. There is no family history of liver disease, although there is a link with diabetes. Alcohol consumption used to be excessive (one bottle of red wine every night) but this has been reduced to about two bottles of wine over the weekend. She is on lisinopril (10 mg/d), sertraline (Lustral), esomeprazole, evening primrose oil and garlic. She has not smoked for 14 years. There is no previous history of high-risk behaviour although she did have a tattoo approximately four years ago.

On examination Ms Marsden is overweight (86 kg). There is no bruising or peripheral oedema. Abdominal examination reveals a palpable edge, but no splenomegaly. Her blood pressure was 162/98. The likely diagnosis is hepatic steatosis (ultrasound). Her cholesterol level is markedly raised (8.4 mmol/l) and she is given ezetimibe (Ezetrol; previous attempts to give a statin worsened liver function). She is referred for optimising her diet to achieve improvement in liver function.

Serum/plasma constituent	Result	Reference range
Albumin (g/l)	47	35–45
Bilirubin (μmol/l)	60	2–17
Cholesterol (mmol/l)	8.4	3.5–7.8
Ferritin (μg/l)	427	10–150 (female)
Glucose (mmol/l)	4.9	3.0–5.0
Haemoglobin (g/dl)	12.2	11.5–15.5 (female)
Iron (μmol/l)	22	10–28 (female)
Potassium (mmol/l)	4.7	3.5–5.0
Sodium (mmol/l)	138	135–150
TIBC (μmol/l)	68	45–72
Total protein (g/l)	74	60–80
Serum/plasma constituent	**Result**	**Reference range**
ALT activity (u/l)	170	10–40
Alkaline phosphatase activity (u/l)	140	40–125
AST activity (u/l)	78	10–34
ESR (mm/hr)	8	<30

Questions to consider

(1) Inspect the clinical chemistry and comment fully on each result, relating this to any disturbed pathophysiology.

(2) The consultant clearly wishes some dietary and lifestyle improvements to assist in improving liver function. What might be an appropriate nutritional care plan for Mrs Marsden?

(3) Consider the client's lifestyle. What particular interventions may assist in bringing her cholesterol down to an interim goal of 6 mmol/l?

(4) Prioritise aspects of Question (3) for attention and list these goals in terms of short- and longer-term goals and say why you have prioritised these in this way.

(5) Suggest ways in which the client's diet can be effectively monitored.

Study questions

(1) Identify the drugs used to treat Mrs Marsden. Write a short account of each of these and explain their mode of action and what they are trying to achieve in this case.

(2) Explain fully the connection between weight and hypertension, and how reducing weight will assist in blood pressure control.

(3) You assess her diet and estimate that her salt intake is about 9 g/d, largely coming from salt added to food and intake of convenience foods. Explain the approach you would use to tackle this during the therapeutic interview. Assume her intake of fruit and vegetables compares favourably with the national average intake.

Case 58 Freda Ingram

Obesity, cognitive behavioural therapy

Study concepts: management of obesity ■ use of a diary in self-monitoring ■ restructuring behaviour to encourage weight loss/maintenance ■ monitoring obese clients

Study context: obesity ■ cognitive behavioural re-structuring

Freda Ingram is a 50-year-old woman who has rheumatoid arthritis and is currently receiving intermittent steroid injections to her lower limbs. Although she is quite mobile, she prefers to drive everywhere in her distinctive little yellow car, recognisable by the sticker in the back windscreen 'I have swum with dolphins in Florida'. She is obese and has struggled to keep her weight down over the past year or so. She eats quite healthily but is a scavenger by nature, preferring to select food from a well-stocked cupboard and her fridge. She finds supermarket shopping quite tiresome, but she does a weekly shop via the Internet. The rest of the time she visits her corner shop before her evening meal and likes to fill her basket with her favourite foods.

Miss Ingram has developed a sweet tooth, which may be as a result of the anti-inflammatory drugs she has been prescribed (sulfasalazine), and following her evening meal she has got into the routine of driving to a petrol station on the pretext of filling the car up with petrol, but instead purchases two to three chocolate bars which she often eats on the way home. Small cream-filled Easter eggs are her favourite, and she does not eat these on the drive home but in front of the television later in the evening. The consultant rheumatologist refers her on for dietary advice. You assess her to be of average height; she refuses to be weighed or have a waist circumference measured.

Questions to consider

(1) You elect to ask Miss Ingram to complete a diet diary prior to coming to the clinic. Comment on this approach, an example of self-monitoring, as a starting point for a therapeutic interview.

(2) You are keen to establish cognitive behaviour restructuring as a way forward in tandem with dietary management. Study the case and identify what behaviours you would want to modify and why.

(3) You estimate that she consumes about 3200 kcal/d, and about a third of this comes from high fat, sweet foods (such as chocolate) and is eaten beyond 9 pm. Discuss the dietary priorities that would be appropriate and outline the short- and longer-term goals.

Study questions

(1) Explain the principles of cognitive behavioural restructuring and the 'readiness to change' model. Discuss the significance of these in the process of managing a client's weight.

(2) Discuss monitoring arrangements that may be appropriate for this, and other clients with a weight problem.

(3) Expand on Question (3) in Questions to consider, to further discuss strategies that may be important in both achieving and sustaining weight loss.

Case 59 Susan O'Connel

Crohn's disease, anorexia

Study concepts: interpretation of clinical chemistry ■ poor dietary intake associated with chronic bowel disease ■ dietary reinforcement over time ■ dietary intake and approaches associated with relapse and remission

Study context: Crohn's disease and associated anorexia nervosa

Susan O'Connel is a young woman (27 years) with an aggressive form of Crohn's disease. She is a long-standing patient of the gastrointestinal unit and has been hospitalised on a number of occasions for resection of her large and small bowel because of adhesions. She is not a very tall girl and currently weighs 41.1 kg, giving her a BMI of 17.1 kg/m². She comes from a broken home although she is very close to her father, with whom she lives. She does very well in hospital, and generally gains weight – with a combination of nocturnal nasogastric feeding together with sip feeds and ordinary hospital diet throughout the day. However, the more often she is hospitalised the less tolerant she becomes of sip feeding.

Susan's periods at home are associated with relapse; her periods of hospitalisation are generally connected with remission and compliance with management. She reports that at home she gets fed up making the huge effort to eat, and simply stops trying. The consultant suspects that she may be anorexic; one of the nurses remarks that she weighed less than an emperor penguin that she saw on a television documentary at the weekend. On Susan's most recent admission, she has the following data recorded as part of routine assessment:

Serum/plasma constituents/parameters	Result	Range
Mid-arm muscle circumference (MAMC) (cm)	19.8 (<25th centile)	50th centile = 21.4
Triceps skinfold thickness (TSF) (mm)	18.1 (>25th centile)	50th centile = 20.0
Albumin (g/l)	22.0	35–45
C-reactive protein (mg/l)	35	<10
Total protein (g/l)	61.4	60–80

The consultant physician requests that the client is fed, as far as possible, with hospital diet and fortified drinks.

Questions to consider

(1) Calculate the patient's nutritional requirements and comment fully on the extent to which you think the client can achieve these through hospital diet food and drink.
(2) What are the nutritional goals for the client both in the short and longer term?
(3) Explain the dietary priorities for this client and using these as a basis for a therapeutic consultation, consider an appropriate approach to deliver this information.
(4) How can nutritional care work towards preventing relapse and establishing a sound nutritional intake in chronic illness?

Study questions

(1) Consider the concentration of C-reactive protein. What is this telling you and how can monitoring this metabolite inform disease activity and therapeutic interventions?
(2) Consider the effect of institutionalisation in this client and explain why this may have a bearing on both her compliance with dietary regimen and her interest in getting better.

Case 60 Dominic Pruz

Ulcerative colitis, loop ileostomy

Study concepts: nutritional status parameters (anthropometry) ■ therapeutic advice to achieve nutritional requirements ■ nutritional goals for ileostomates ■ formulating dietary advice ■ managing disinterest in food

Study context: loop ileostomy and weight loss

Dominic Pruz is a 41-year-old Baptist minister who evangelises in a small village church in rural England. He lives in the manse with his wife and four children under the age of 10 years. He has a long history of ulcerative colitis, and this has been managed for some years with a combination of steroid therapy, anti-inflammatory drugs and diet. He reports that he has been 'through the mill', diet-wise, having been on a dairy-free diet, an elimination diet and endless combinations of sip feeds. He enjoyed some long spells of remission but his general health has begun to deteriorate and his appetite has been poor. He has lost faith in the positive effects of dietary management.

Dr Pruz has recently returned from a visit to his homeland in Zimbabwe, where a pan-proctocolectomy was performed. He had a loop ileostomy placed and stoma formed, and has been described by his consultant as a 'bag loser', as effluent pours through the stoma. He has been plagued with intermittent bowel symptoms ever since (abdominal discomfort and pain, bloating and flatulence). He has lost about 16 kg over the past 18 months. His height is 1.74 m and he currently weighs 73 kg. He has nausea most of the time and has lost interest in food. He is seen by his consultant. Routine blood work and nutritional assessment reveals the following clinical information:

Serum/plasma constituents/ parameters	Result	Range
Mid-arm muscle circumference (MAMC) (cm)	21.4 (<50th centile)	50th centile = 22.0
Triceps skinfold thickness (TSF) (mm)	22.1 (<50th centile)	50th centile = 23.0
Total protein (g/l)	67.3	60–80
Albumin (g/l)	31.0	35–45
Haemoglobin (g/dl)	8.9	11.5–15.5 (male)
Folate (ng/ml)	3.9	>5
Potassium (mmol/l)	2.2	3.5–5.0
Sodium (mmol/l)	130	135–150

Questions to consider

(1) Investigate the rationale for the various dietary interventions experienced by Dr Pruz, including the dairy product-free diet and the elimination diet. Consider also the weight of evidence supporting the use of these in the conservative management of ulcerative colitis.

(2) Consider the blood investigations, and taking each parameter in turn, indicate the possible implications of these for baseline nutritional status and for future nutritional strategy.

(3) Discuss the objectives of dietary management and prioritise nutritional goals for Dr Pruz.

(4) Calculate his main nutritional requirements and interpret these into a practical plan of action for the client.

(5) Discuss suitable monitoring arrangements to assist in determining whether the client is achieving his goals.

Study questions

(1) Construct a simple, but explicit information sheet for a client with ileostomy and pouch. Use two columns to indicate both the dietary objective together with some reasoning.

(2) Explain the relationship with anaemia and anorexia in a client of this type.

(3) This patient has lost interest (or faith) in food and is unconvinced of the role that diet plays in quality of life. With this in mind, discuss the approach that may be taken to motivate the client to better place diet in the context of his health.

Case 61 Rudi Jordache

Obesity, behaviour modification

Study concepts: eating associated with constant access to inappropriate foods ■ dietary intake associated with inappropriate behaviours ■ opportunity for lifestyle interventions ■ motivational and compliance issues

Study context: obesity ■ behavioural modification and lifestyle intervention

Rudi Jordache is a 58-year-old restauranteur originally from a small town on the Austrian/Italian border. His restaurant has a distinctly Italian influence and it has recently been awarded a prestigious Michelin star. He prides himself in his selection of eclectic menu items; his variety of cold Italian meats and antipasto is renowned.

He has recently been struggling a bit with his health. He has suffered spontaneous rib fractures as a result of osteopenia, for which he is taking Adcal. He has now got osteoarthritis of both knees which is severely limiting his mobility.

He currently weighs 109 kg (1.74 m) and has gained 10 kg in the past year following cessation of smoking after a health scare. He has a waist circumference of 114 cm. He insists on eating a main meal (18.00 hr) with his staff, but unfortunately retreats to his flat later in the evening (20.00 hr) and consumes a substantial snack of salami or Parma ham, garlic sausage and Italian bread. He confesses to *swallowing food whole*, and swipes food from the cold table when he passes at lunch time (he can eat as many as 10–12 slices salami). He is *hooked on salt*. He has no breakfast.

During his days off, he surrounds himself with food and does little but sit in his chair watching old movies, or cricket on television whilst eating and drinking his favourite German beer.

Questions to consider

(1) Assess the client's health risk in relation to his lifestyle and diet.
(2) Consider what might be appropriate intervention in relation to Question (1) and explain the rationale for your consideration.
(3) Comment on the ability and likely adherence of the client to adopt the intervention strategy explained in Question (2).
(4) Clearly the client has constant access to food. How might any therapeutic interview attempt to bring this into the equation?
(5) Calculate the energy content of a suitable intervention diet to induce slow and gradual weight loss over time.
(6) Interpret the energy prescription into a suitable daily diet pattern for the client.
(7) The client shows up for his second face-to-face consultation (10 weeks from baseline), having failed to attend the previous two appointments made for him. His waist circumference is 108 cm and he has managed to do a little walking since last time, although his dietary pattern remains unchanged. Consider the approach that may be taken.

Study questions

(1) Consider fully the opportunity to motivate a client such as this and explain how this might achieve some improvement in achieving even a short-term goal.
(2) A client with low physical activity presents a significant challenge. What strategies might be important to consider when managing a client like this?
(3) Explain the relationship between waist circumference, BMI and associated health risk.
(4) Explain the possible implications of a patient's compliance with a poor history of clinic attendance.

Cases

(5) What alternative strategies, apart from one-to-one counselling, might be considered in inducing weight loss and lifestyle change and then maintaining weight loss and what is the evidence supporting or refuting these ideas?

(6) Explain the association between weight maintenance and smoking.

Case 62 Glenda Henderson

Gestational diabetes, obesity

Study concepts: dietary intake associated with family priorities ■ managing a diet to reduce risk of cardiovascular disease and diabetes ■ motivational and compliance issues associated with overweight ■ behavioural modification and lifestyle intervention

Study context: gestational diabetes ■ obesity

Glenda Henderson is a 44-year-old woman who delivered twin sons (first confinement) about 14 months ago. She received pre-conceptual advice, partly informed by a strong family history of diabetes; her mother has type 2 diabetes and her older sister has type 1 diabetes. She was given help in managing her diet pre-conceptually; she was slightly overweight at that time.

Glenda's confinement was perfectly uneventful, except that she had two routine fasting blood glucose tests of 6.1 mmol/l and 6.8 mmol/l at around 26 weeks of the pregnancy. She delivered at 35 weeks of the pregnancy. Her blood glucose control has been assessed by her GP in the recent past; all tests were normal.

Her current weight is 97.5 kg (height 1.77 m) and she is normotensive (105/60 mmHg). She is shortly to have a health screen for cholesterol. She is keen to reduce her risk of developing diabetes in the longer term. She finds looking after the twins demanding and whilst she plans their dietary intakes carefully, she pays less attention to herself and tends to snack on foods rejected by the boys.

Her life is built around the routine of managing her children and looking after the house. She has a puppy (cocker spaniel) which she takes for walks twice each day.

Questions to consider

(1) Assuming this client was referred to you for general advice at the booking stage, what might that information consist of, and why?

(2) Assuming you see this woman at 26 weeks' gestation, with regard to her weight and blood sugars, what would be the focus of any therapeutic counselling and why?

(3) Using the general advice given in the answer to Question (1), what particular aspects might be useful to reinforce for this client, and why?

(4) You investigate the pattern of weight gain in this client, and discover that most of the gains were associated with dietary discrepancies at about 14 or 15 weeks' gestation. This was associated with getting over the sickly phase and consuming lots of salty and sugary foods. Her dietary pattern has levelled out, although there is still a tendency to eat these foods, perhaps elevated from baseline and more than the national average. What advice would you give and how can you convince the client of its benefit?

(5) What particular lifestyle interventions would you especially promote and why?

(6) She arrives at clinic for routine assessment. She presents for dietary advice – explain her longer-term nutritional goals and suggest how these will be monitored.

(7) Talk through the dietary advice you would give, carefully prioritising the information. Give the basis for your prioritisation.

Study questions

(1) Consider and discuss the approaches taken in the management of pregnancy in terms of optimal weight. How is weight gain monitored and assessed?

(2) Investigate the likely focus of any pre-conceptual advice given to any couples planning pregnancies. How much of this is diet and lifestyle focused?

(3) Consider the evidence that recommends dietary intervention in the care of a client with gestational diabetes. Classify the various recommendations into priorities and explain how these may be included into a therapeutic dietary consultation.

(4) Explain the association between obesity and impaired glucose tolerance. Assuming that any dietary intervention planned for this client group might include some counselling on the concept of glycaemic index, explain the concept and explain how this may inform dietary advice given, and the approach taken, in a therapeutic interview.

Case 63 Daniel Borden
Head injury, nutritional support

Study concepts: assessing nutritional requirements in a head-injured patient ■ establishing aggressive nutritional support ■ monitoring arrangements in head-injured patients ■ transition from nasogastric feeding to hospital diet

Study context: head injury ■ nutritional support

Daniel Borden is a 39-year-old family man who was painting the outside of his house, No. 32, Chesapeake Close. As he was stretching to paint under the eaves he fell from his ladder onto the concrete patio below, where he lay unconscious for about an hour until found by his neighbour. He was rushed to the accident and emergency unit where he presented with a 15 cm deep laceration to his scalp together with two fractured ribs and head and neck bruising. His admission weight was 83 kg (1.75 m) and his intra-cranial pressure was normal.

At 48 hours post-injury Mr Borden's intra-cranial pressure began to rise and cerebral oedema caused an increase in seizure activity managed by barbiturate therapy. He is mechanically ventilated and remains under moderate to heavy sedation in the high dependency unit.

Questions to consider

(1) Assuming Mr Borden has no significant medical history, calculate his main nutritional requirements and decide, with a justified rationale, the route of administration of nutritional support.
(2) Explain the nutritional goals for this patient in the short term and discuss the monitoring arrangements that may assist in evaluating his progress.
(3) Ten days post-injury the patient begins to respond, intra-cranial pressure returns to normal and he regains a fully conscious, but sleepy state. Discuss how his nutritional priorities may change in terms of forward planning.
(4) At day 14, Mr Borden is sitting up in a general medical ward and deemed ready to start oral diet. Explain how this may be started and discuss the approaches, including monitoring, that may be taken as recovery, and hence oral intake proceeds.

Study questions

(1) Explain any special arrangements that may be built into care planning should the patient not respond and remain unconscious in the longer term.
(2) Explain the significance of a rise in ICP and how this might be managed and monitored medically.

Case 64 Shaun Gascoine

Oesophageal carcinoma

Study concepts: progressive dysphagia ■ management of weight loss ■ maintenance of weight during aggressive cancer therapy ■ discharge arrangements including nutritional care

Study context: oesophageal carcinoma ■ nutritional support

Shaun Gascoine (aged 62 years of age) is a retired head teacher of a local primary school. Now that he has a bit more free time, he is spending more quality time with his grandchildren. He has also enrolled on a couple of night classes at a community college (Italian cooking and conversational French) to keep himself busy. Lately, he has been feeling tired and off his food, but put this down to getting older and needing to wind down from his professional life.

Mr Gascoine is 179.9 cm and 68.2 kg and presents to his family doctor with a six-month history of progressive dysphagia. He manages to drink quite well but has noticed some difficulty swallowing bread, meat (unless it is very tender) and biscuits. He reckons he has lost about a stone since Christmas (three months ago). His serum albumin is 29 g/l; his MAMC and TSF measurements are within the 25–50th centiles.

Oesophageal cancer is diagnosed, but the prognosis is good (no obvious lymph node involvement). The treatment plan is for aggressive radiation therapy (four weeks), to start as soon as possible, followed by oesophago-gastrectomy and prophylactic chemotherapy (four to six weeks).

Questions to consider

(1)   Consider the nutritional priorities for this patient at baseline (i.e. before radiotherapy begins), during radiotherapy, following surgery and during chemotherapy.
(2)   Calculate his nutritional requirements at each stage of treatment, assuming his weight is the same (i.e. that he is able to sustain his presenting weight).
(3)   Explain how it may be anticipated that Mr Gascoine achieves his nutritional requirements, assuming that he is nauseous following therapy.
(4)   Discuss discharge arrangements to include nutritional intake and monitoring.

Study questions

(1)   In a client with upper gastrointestinal cancer, explain why a prognosis may be judged as good or bad. What might the tell-tale signs be?
(2)   List the major side-effects of both chemo- and radiotherapy and how these may be ameliorated via dietary management.

Case 65 Frank Calder

Type 1 diabetes, overweight

Study concepts: interpretation of dietary assessment ■ therapeutic dietary issues ■ justification of method of dietary and eating assessment ■ forming a clinical decision

Study context: overweight with type 1 diabetes

Frank Calder has been a diabetic for some considerable time and remains
on insulin (short-acting prior to each meal) at the age of 70 years. He has
been lost to follow-up for the past 10 years or so, partly because he has
been moving around a lot, and partly because he is a retired general practitioner and believes he can adequately self-monitor. He is quite strong-
willed and independent.

Mr Calder was recently planting a row of new potatoes, when he slipped
and fractured his left hip. He maintains that he manages his diet perfectly,
and that his weight never fluctuates (BMI of 27 kg/m²). At history, it is
revealed that he relies heavily on convenience foods (especially since the
death of his partner), using whatever portion comes in a packet or a box,
yet he is meticulous about monitoring his fruit and vegetable intake (half a
banana; half a glass of fruit juice). He enjoys nothing better at the weekends
(and sometimes during the week) than driving to the Orient Express, which
is an express food bar specialising in Chinese foods.

The admitting physician refers the client for a diabetic review and he
attends diabetic clinic some six weeks after the fall. Clinical information
documented in his case notes is as follows:

'Well-nourished' and 'florid' and 'feels well'
BP 170/80
Blood glucose slightly elevated
HbA₁c 12%
Traces of glucose in urine
Blood glucose tests for past 9 months records (4.5–6.7 mmol/l)

Questions to consider

(1) A rough dietary assessment reveals a daily intake of about 2400 kcal,
90 g protein and about 37% of the client's total energy coming from
fat. Explain any potential improvements to his intake that may assist his
diabetic control and general health.

(2) Consider the lifestyle issues that may be discussed during the first consultation and explain fully the nature of these and the evidence that
suggests that these are beneficial to the diabetic state.

(3) Explain the nature of dietary reinforcement that may be given to this client, given his high level of independency from the diabetic clinic.

(4) Consider the methods of evaluation that may be useful to monitor this client over time and explain what information they would give.

Study questions

(1) Explain the purpose of measuring glycated haemoglobin as a means of testing compliance with diabetic instruction.

(2) What are the main indicators to determine whether a diabetic client can be considered to be stable?

(3) What are the principal clinical outcomes for the management of the diabetic client?

(4) What are the short- and longer-term nutritional goals associated with the care of a diabetic client?

(5) Sketch out a care pathway for the management of a diabetic client to indicate the role and engagement of the other healthcare professionals associated with the care of a diabetic subject.

(6) Explain the main complications that are associated with poor diabetic control.

Case 66 Stanislaw Roza

Hypertension, ethnic diet, health risk

Study concepts: traditional Polish diet and health risk implications ■ potential and feasible dietary and lifestyle interventions ■ shifting dietary emphasis in an ethnic diet

Study context: hypertension and health risk associated with ethnic diet and culture

Stanislaw (pronounced Stanislav) Roza is a Polish immigrant worker (aged 28 years) who arrived in the UK a few months ago with his wife Ania and plans to settle in Inverness where the eastern European migrant community forms the second largest ethnic group. Although fairly well educated, he has recently obtained work in a factory which processes smoked fish products. He regularly visits a local Polish bread shop and delicatessen to purchase familiar Polish foods.

Mr Roza remains loyal to his traditional eating pattern: a cooked breakfast (including croissants served with honey), a full lunch (a large bowl of hearty cabbage soup, or *bigos* – a sauerkraut and meat stew, served with dark rye bread) and an early evening meal (4 pm) consisting of fried blood sausage (made with *kasza* or buckwheat, lard and onions), potato dumplings (*pyzy*) served with sour cream and a vegetable (cucumbers, pickles or courgettes). The meal is always finished with a slice of *makowiec* (poppyseed cake) or *sernik* (cheesecake). Later in the evening he sits down to have a snack of *halva*, and sometimes *faworki* (pork crackling) with Polish beer (strong). He enjoys a good measure of Polish vodka (40% alcohol) served neat.

Mr Roza cycles to work and is a non-smoker. As part of an occupational health screen, he is found to have a somewhat elevated blood pressure (190/88 mmHg) and is slightly overweight (waist circumference 98 cm). He is referred for lifestyle advice.

Questions to consider

(1) Explain the possible line of enquiry that might be taken in a consultation with the client to ascertain potential sources of weakness in the client's diet and lifestyle in terms of health risk.

(2) Eyeball the references to food intake. What assumptions or implications have these for health risk and poor blood pressure control?

(3) Consider the probable diet and lifestyle interventions that may assist in general improvement in health as well as control of blood pressure.

(4) Explain any particular approaches that might be taken if the client wishes to cling to traditional foods and meal patterns.

Case 67 Peter Donnelly

Overweight, hypertension

Study concepts: interpretation of dietary assessment ■ therapeutic dietary issues ■ justification of method of dietary and eating assessment ■ forming a clinical decision

Study context: overweight ■ hypertension

Peter Donnelly is 35 years of age. He is unemployed, and has been for many years, essentially because of long-term mental health issues. He is unable to cope with the routine demands of a job and currently receives unemployment benefit together with a small disability allowance. He lives in a small flat and lies in bed most days until about 11.00 or 12.00 hr. He has little incentive to get out and about, although recently he has taken up swimming. He lives on his own with two cats (Cajun and Cormack) for company.

Over the past few years Mr Donnelly has lost interest in himself; he looks dirty and is unshaven and has put on quite a bit of weight (current weight is 13 stone, 5 ft 9 in). He smokes 20 cigarettes each day and uses recreational drugs. His alcohol consumption is probably high (>4 units/d) and he meets friends occasionally in a local bar. He has a history of self-harming.

He recently attended the hospital to have his drugs reviewed (anti-depressants (Prozac) and mood stabilisers) and the consultant took his blood pressure (195/98). A casual conversation about his diet suggested that his salt intake may be high and contributing to poor control of blood pressure.

Day 1	Day 2	Day 3
Late breakfast	**Late breakfast**	**Late breakfast**
Crunchy maple and pecan cereal with semi-skimmed milk Tea with milk and sugar	2 crunchy cereal bars Tea with milk and sugar	Bran flakes and sultana cereal with semi-skimmed milk Tea with milk and sugar
2 pm lunch	**2 pm lunch**	**2 pm lunch**
'Meal Deal' – white bread sandwich with tuna mayonnaise and salad, packet of crisps, cream cheese dip (breadsticks) Blackcurrant squash	2 slices white toast, spread with Marmite and butter Glass of semi-skimmed milk Apple	2 slices white toast with butter and two good-size chunks cheddar cheese Orange squash
6.30 pm evening meal	**6.30 pm evening meal**	**6.30 pm evening meal**
Bowl of pasta with green pesto sauce, 2 slices garlic bread and 2 glasses cheap red wine	Cottage pie with extra serving of chips, Glass of cider Half chocolate bar	Left over cottage pie with box meal (haddock and chips), Glass of cider

Questions to consider

(1) Look at the three-day dietary record and classify the intakes into whether you think they show low, medium or high intakes of dietary sodium, as compared with usual UK intakes.
(2) Calculate accurately the salt (sodium) and energy intake and compare these against reference usual consumption standards. Explain what this tells you.
(3) Comment fully on how the intakes compare with target recommendations for this client.
(4) Explain the dietary improvements that the client might make to reduce salt (sodium) intake to assist blood pressure control.
(5) Consider the changes to lifestyle that the client may benefit from in terms of overall health.

Study questions

(1) Explain the relationship between salt and sodium when assessing a client's intake.
(2) Explain the practical advice that might be given to a client to reduce his exposure to dietary sodium.

Case 68 John Mortimer

Stroke

Study concepts: diet implications in cause of stroke ■ lifestyle issues ■ management of a client through rehabilitation ■ multi-disciplinary teamwork ■ longer-term diet management

Study context: stroke

John Mortimer, aged 58 years and a judge, drove to work as usual. He was found, slumped at his desk, in the middle of the morning by a colleague who immediately called for an ambulance. He was taken to the accident and emergency department in an unconscious state. He regained consciousness within an hour but was confused, disorientated and frightened.

On examination Mr Mortimer weighed 120.4 kg (171 cm), had a pulse rate of 140 beats per minute and a blood pressure of 220/110. After a further series of tests he was diagnosed with a cerebral haemorrhage from the left cerebral artery with associated right-sided paralysis. He was aphasic.

Mr Mortimer progressed from clear liquids to a soft hospital diet. Within three weeks he was able to tolerate a full hospital diet, with assistance from the occupational therapist and dietitian. He was later referred to a speech and language therapist and physiotherapist for assessment and rehabilitation. Within four months he was back at home and managing to walk with a stick. He complied with most of the rehabilitation exercises at home.

Questions to consider

(1) Explain the management objectives of the client at the point of care (i.e. at the hospital following initial assessment).
(2) Considering the physical data given in this case, what might be the short-term nutritional goals for Mr Mortimer and how will these be achieved and monitored in the ward following admission?
(3) As the client progressed to becoming a much less-dependent eater (at about three weeks' post-stroke) how will the nutritional priorities change and what might be the longer-term objectives for nutritional management?
(4) Indicate what you think might be useful discharge planning objectives for Mr Mortimer and propose how clinical outcomes can be monitored.

Study questions

(1) Review the causes of stroke, highlighting the physiological mechanisms that influence aetiology.

(2) Examine the evidence that diet intake and lifestyle may influence the risk of developing stroke and explain the population-wide strategy to reduce incidence of stroke and other chronic diseases associated with faulty diet/overnutrition.

(3) Whilst the client's total serum cholesterol level is not given, if one assumes that it may be elevated, what particular dietary/lifestyle interventions may assist in reducing a high level?

(4) Comment fully on the role and function of the MDT approach in the care of stroke clients.

Case 69 Maude Ashby

Stroke, clinical chemistry

Study concepts: dietary intervention post-stroke ■ clinical chemistry as a basis for feeding ■ management of a client using nasogastric feeding ■ re-feeding syndrome

Study context: stroke ■ clinical chemistry

Maude Ashby lives on her own and remains fiercely independent despite her years (80 years of age). She returned from a recent trip to the local shops to collect her pension and do a bit of grocery shopping and shortly after this collapsed on her kitchen floor. Her daughter visited her the following morning and called 999 to get help. Mrs Ashby was immediately transported to the local district hospital. It was estimated that she had been unconscious for about 16 hours. She has a stable weight (62 kg, height 160 cm).

On admission, the consultant diagnosed a stroke and routine blood investigations were done and repeated (24-hr post-admission). The results are given below. She remains on intra-venous fluids for four days, and following the unsafe swallow assessment by the SLT, the decision is made to feed using a nasogastric feed.

Serum/plasma constituent	Result (on admission)	Result (at 1 day post-admission)	Reference range
Albumin (g/l)	45	41	35–45
Calcium (mmol/l)	2.5	2.4	2.25–2.65
C-reactive protein (mg/l)	7	7	<10
Creatinine (µmol/l)	136	126	40–130
Haemoglobin (g/dl)	13.1	12.5	11.5–15.5 (female)
Magnesium (mmol/l)	0.7	0.8	0.7–1.0
Potassium (mmol/l)	4.9	4.1	3.5–5.0
Phosphate (mmol/l)	1.4	0.9	0.8–1.4
Total protein (g/l)	72	69	60–80

Cases

Questions to consider

(1) Taking each constituent in turn, comment on the patient's clinical chemistry results on admission.

(2) Comment fully on the patient's clinical chemistry on admission + day 1 and explain the changes.

(3) In addition to blood tests, what other clinical information might be useful to assist with interpretation of the results?

(4) The patient is to start nasogastric feeding. Indicate and explain the blood tests you would request prior to feeding.

(5) Discuss the nutritional care plan for this client and relate this to Question (3).

(6) Calculate the patient's fluid and electrolyte requirements (calcium, sodium, magnesium, phosphate and potassium).

(7) Using a standard feed, design a possible feeding regimen.

Study questions

(1) Explain the possible causes of dehydration in an older, but free-living individual.

(2) Describe the possible bedside observations that may assist in classifying an individual as dehydrated.

(3) Explain the possible influence of dehydration when interpreting clinical chemistry results.

(4) Explain the phenomenon known as 're-feeding syndrome', and discuss how this can be avoided in clinical practice.

Case 70 Christopher Smith

Terminal cancer, palliative care

Study concepts: nutritional considerations in palliative care ■ meeting nutritional requirements on hospital diet ■ diet priorities in a patient with poor prognosis ■ ethical issues surrounding nutritional support

Study context: advanced cancer ■ palliative care

Christopher Smith was born in the early 1950s and was recently admitted to hospital for investigation of abdominal pain and weight loss. Following a laparotomy, a differentiated carcinoma was found and considered by the surgeon to be inoperable. The client's prognosis is poor and the discharge plan includes hospice/palliative care. The patient is referred to the dietitian seven days following surgery.

The patient weighs 52 kg (1.75 m) and has lost 12 kg over the past three months. He remains cheerful and is tolerating hospital diet quite well, although he is complaining about the taste of some of the sip feeds.

Questions to consider

(1) Advocate the short-term nutritional goals for the patient and consider how these can be achieved using hospital diet and sip feeds.

(2) The client is referred some seven days following surgery. Discuss the ethics of the referral time frame in this case and the apparent absence of nutritional screening.

(3) Calculate the major nutritional requirements for this patient and comment fully on the extent to which hospital diet might provide these both now, and in the longer term.

(4) Comment on the extent to which you consider how aggressive nutritional support should be in this case.

(5) Recommend and explain how the patient's progress may be monitored.

(6) Construct possible virtual discharge planning advice for the hospice aftercare.

Study questions

(1) Explain the ethics of feeding a terminally ill patient and the extent to which you think nutritional support should meet nutritional requirements.

(2) Assuming the patient cannot meet all nutritional requirements, what may be the diet priorities for a client who is to receive palliative care?

(3) Discuss how a residential care home or hospice may be assisted to deliver a given level of nutritional care.

The diaries
(and contexts)

Diary 1 Weight loss, diet patterns

The diary of a man (aged 45 years) with weight loss and an insecure diagnosis

Nicholas Guest is a recruitment consultant who commutes to Edinburgh and Glasgow from his home in the Scottish borders. He has been experiencing a change in bowel habits with associated weight loss and was referred to a consultant physician for investigations. A colonoscopy revealed no mucosal abnormality, indicating that the patient's minor rectal bleeding was suspected as innocent. He has long-standing bronchitis for which he is being treated with bronchodilators (via a nasal spray). Three years ago, he weighed 11.5 stone; at clinic today he weighs 57 kg. He is anaemic, and regularly takes part in 10 km runs.

Further tests revealed a worm in the caecum, almost certainly a threadworm and a single treatment of 100 mg mebendazole was recommended. The consultant was unsure whether the presence of a worm(s) was relevant to the weight loss and asked for a full dietary assessment.

A typical daily dietary pattern for Mr Guest is as follows: he works in Glasgow for three days and Edinburgh for two days. Weekends follow the Edinburgh pattern and include 2 units of alcohol.

	Edinburgh		Glasgow
Breakfast (at home)	Small bowl of porridge, made with 250 ml skimmed milk Cup of tea (30 ml semi-skimmed milk)	**Breakfast** (on train)	2 bacon rolls 2 cups of tea with whole milk
am	Cup of tea (30 ml semi-skimmed milk)	**am** (at office)	Cup of tea with milk (from vending machine)
Lunch (at office)	500 ml natural yoghurt 2 green apples	**Lunch** (in shopping mall)	Bowl of light pasta or sushi Large glass Chablis
pm	Cup of tea (30 ml semi-skimmed milk)	**pm** (at office)	2 or 3 sausage rolls 2 green apples
Evening meal (at home)	200 g melon, 100 g grapes 100 g chicken or lean meat as risotto or bolognese 100 g plain boiled vegetables	**pm** (on train)	3 chocolate cup cakes Cup of tea with milk
Supper	Cup of peppermint tea	**Evening meal** (at home) **Supper**	As Edinburgh Cup of peppermint tea

Diaries

Questions to consider

(1) Assuming that the two extracts from Mr Guest's diaries represent typical and habitual dietary intakes over the working week, what conclusions may be drawn from the intakes in terms of dietary patterns, quantitative and qualitative nutrient content?

(2) Study the two intakes, and using your knowledge of food constituents, assess them in terms of protein and energy content. How near do you think these will achieve recommendations for the client?

(3) Now calculate the menus using a food/nutrient database and compare the totals for protein and energy intake with your 'eyeball' (look and see) assessment in (2). What does this tell you about your accuracy and what might be a useful action plan to become more confident in making eyeball judgements?

(4) Comment on the extent to which food selection is governed by day-to-day circumstances.

(5) Draft a letter to the consultant, framing the main findings of the diaries in the context of weight loss and dietary patterning.

(6) Outline the advice that may be advocated for Mr Guest given his circumstances and personal food preferences.

Study questions

(1) Explore the potential impact of dietary patterns (meal frequency, intake of snack foods and timing of meals) on weight maintenance.

(2) What does the evidence suggest about eating behaviour in relation to general health?

(3) What might be the potential consequences for health of eating food quickly and rushing meals?

(4) What practical dietary instructions might be given to a client to slow food ingestion?

Diary 2 Migraine, diet exclusion

The diary of a young woman (aged 25 years) with a life-long history of migraine

Episodes of migraine have exacerbated since the birth of her son (some 18 months ago). The main concern is her heavy dependence on medication whilst attempting a second pregnancy. Her consultant is keen to explore elimination of likely migraine trigger foods/drinks from her diet. She reports that she has a 'permanent headache with bad ones most evenings'.

	Day 1	Day 2
Breakfast	Small bowl of bran flakes with enough semi-skimmed milk to dampen Slice of wholemeal bread with butter and strawberry jam Cup of decaffeinated milky coffee	Small bowl of bran flakes with enough semi-skimmed milk to dampen Slice of wholemeal bread with butter and chocolate spread Cup of decaffeinated milky coffee
am	Water 1 doughnut	Water, Half a slice of lemon meringue pie Half a slice of white toast with butter
Lunch	Half a melon Chicken sandwich on brown bread 5 cherry tomatoes Watercress, small handful Grapes, strawberries, pineapple Glass of red wine	Water Seeded bagel with smoked salmon and low fat mayonnaise 3 mini-chocolate crispy cakes 4 small cream-filled chocolate eggs Glass of Chardonnay
pm (17.30 hr)	Mug of decaffeinated cappuccino Chocolate/mint biscuit bar	Half ice-cream cone (from baby) 2 mini-chocolate crisy cake
pm (19.30 hr)	3 breadsticks Apple 2 dessertspoons leftover baked beans 2 slices soda bread and butter	Dessertspoon leftover rice 6 black olives (in oil) Water
Evening meal (20.00 hr)	Portion baked chicken in oat crust Hot lentils with onion, goat's cheese, roasted vegetables: courgettes, fennel, onion, peppers, and tomato with balsamic vinegar and oil Milk chocolate 'bunny' Cup decaffeinated milky coffee	Half melon Spaghetti bolognese, made with minced beef, onions, mushrooms, peppers, tomatoes and herbs Vanilla ice-cream cone Double chocolate cookie Mug of decaffeinated milky coffee Glass of red wine
Supper	Nil	Piece of bitter chocolate

Questions to consider

(1) Inspect the diary entries and comment on the balance and likely dietary exposure to agents implicated in the aetiology of migraines.

(2) Assuming these two excerpts from a seven-day diary are typical of her intake, discuss your findings with a view to formulating appropriate dietary advice for the client.

(3) Comment fully on the pathophysiology and evidence on which any advice may be based in order to decrease the risk of migraines.

Diary 3 Type 2 diabetes, diverticulitis

The diary of a woman (aged 55 years) with a history of diverticulitis

This lady is a little overweight and has type 2 diabetes. She is referred for dietary review following laparoscopy and the diagnosis of diverticulitis. Her condition has settled with antibiotic therapy, but her consultant is keen to manage her health by dietary means. She is not very active and has diarrhoea (two to three episodes per day) interspersed with constipation. She is a former 'slimmer of the year'.

	Day 1	Day 2
Breakfast	[Mug of tea with milk on rising] Porridge made with water Skimmed milk poured over	[Mug of tea with milk on rising] Porridge made with water Skimmed milk poured over
am	Mug of tea with semi-skimmed milk Cheese scone with butter	Glass of vegetable juice
Lunch	1 grilled pork sausage 2 grilled rashers back bacon One slice of white bread with butter Dry fried egg and grilled tomato Mug of tea with semi-skimmed milk	Small bowl of pea soup One slice of white bread toasted 3oz sardines in tomato sauce Small salad (tomato, onion, lettuce)
pm (13.30 hr)	Glass of low calorie bitter lemon drink	Green apple
pm (14.30 hr)	Small plate of lentil and ham soup (sweet potato and butternut squash added)	4 rice cakes
pm (16.45 hr)	Green apple Mug of tea with semi-skimmed milk	
Evening meal (19.15 hr)	5 green olives 6 oz roast chicken (skin removed) 5 oz roast potatoes (no fat) Broccoli and carrots Tablespoon hot pepper sauce	6 oz grilled sirloin 5 oz salad potatoes Salad (peppers, red onion, cherry tomatoes, lettuce)
Supper	2 glasses of low calorie lemonade Half pint of skimmed milk to drink	Small piece home-made sponge cake Half pint of skimmed milk to drink

Questions to consider

(1)   Inspect the diary entries and comment on the quantitative and qualitative balance or shape of the intake.

(2)   Comment on the specific areas of investigation that may be appropriate to explore in light of the client's diagnosis.

(3)   Assuming these two excerpts from a seven-day diary are typical of her intake, discuss your findings with a view to formulating appropriate dietary advice for the client.

(4)   Explain what you consider to be important lifestyle priorities for the client to adopt to assist with general health as well as her diagnoses.

Diary 4 Irritable bowel syndrome

The diary of a young woman (aged 21 years) with a history of irritable bowel syndrome

This drama student has a normal BMI ($21.7 \, \text{kg/m}^2$) and is referred for dietary advice. She has upper abdominal symptoms including functional dyspepsia, bloating and nausea together with diarrhoea (which she reports stems from intake of bread, pasta, spicy and dairy foods). She has a diagnosis of abdominal migraine, has become disengaged from her social life and does not do any exercise.

Saturday	Sunday
2 pm Baked potato, butter and cheese Glass lemonade	**2 pm** Cheese sandwich Glass of orange juice topped up with lemonade
6 pm Take-away meal: Chicken tikka masala Pilau rice	**7 pm** Take-away meal: Sticky chilli chicken Egg fried rice
11 pm Packet of crisps Glass of lemonade	**10 pm** Packet of crisps Glass of lemonade

Monday	Tuesday
4 pm Packet of salt-and-vinegar crisps	**12 pm** 3 chicken spring rolls
7 pm Large serving of macaroni and cheese (box from the supermarket to serve two)	**10 pm** Large serving cheesy pasta
11 pm Chocolate trifle	**11 pm** 2 glasses wine (working on an essay)
	1 am Packet of crisps 1 glass wine

Questions to consider

(1) Inspect the diary entries and comment on the quantitative and qualitative balance or shape of the intake.

(2) The client also notes symptoms of bloating, arising progressively throughout each day and peaking at about 8 pm. Explain how her dietary intake may be restructured to reduce the risks of development of her global symptoms.

(3) Summarise the main dietary agents and behaviours associated with irritable bowel syndrome and explain how these influence the therapeutic approach in this client.

Diary 5 Coronary artery disease, health risk

The diary of an older woman (aged 70 years) with a history of coronary atheroma

This thin woman has familial hypercholesterolaemia. Her annual blood work reveals a total cholesterol concentration of 3.8 mmol/l with an LDL level of 2.3 mmol/l. Her consultant wants to reduce her total cholesterol level to below 2.5 mmol/l. The patient sends a dietary record ahead of her consultation. She is taking statins.

	Day 1	Subsequent days
Breakfast	40 g porridge made with water 10 g oat bran 150 ml soya milk 200 ml red tea, no milk	• Intakes are similar, except she varies the main course major protein sources (she has lean sirloin steak, tuna, cottage cheese, and so on). The timing of her meals and snacks are carefully managed (by the clock).
am	200 ml red tea, no milk 20 g pumpkin seeds 90 g peeled apple	

Lunch	100 g canned salmon, drained
	45 g cherry tomatoes
	180 g boiled, salad potatoes
	150 g natural yoghurt, sprinkled with 5 g linseeds and 10 g split almonds
		• In addition to her dietary intake, she takes the following supplements:
		  • *For liver cleansing*: 20 g lime juice made up with water, apple cider, 5 g honey and malt vinegar to 200 ml
		  • *For osteoporosis* (never diagnosed): 500 mg calcium citrate

pm	200 ml hot water with 10 g vegetable extract and malt	

Diaries

	Day 1	Subsequent days
Evening meal	*75 g roast chicken, no skin* *75 g boiled broccoli* *100 g boiled carrot, sprinkled with* *pine nut kernels* *100 ml dry white wine*	● *For restless legs*: vitamin B$_{12}$, folic acid, magnesium, iron, zinc and selenium supplement, garlic ● *For tiredness*: additional iron tonic and multivitamin B supplement
Supper	*30 g tropical fruit and nut* *mixture* *2 cracker biscuits with* *5 g vegetable extract spread* *50 ml whole milk to drink*	● *For the heart*: hawthorn tincture

Diaries

Questions to consider

(1) Inspect the diary entry and comment on the general pattern of the intake.

(2) The intake is estimated to contain about 1300 kcal/d. Assess the intake in terms of cardiovascular risk or health, explaining your reasoning fully.

(3) Identify with reasoning, the main issues that may be explored with the client in terms of her usual diet and possible modification to achieve the new clinical goal of a total cholesterol concentration of <2 mmol/l.

(4) Comment fully on the rationale and likely benefit (or otherwise) of the supplements taken routinely and indicate how mention of these might occur in the course of the therapeutic interview.

Diary 6 Hypertension, renal calculi

The diary of a man (aged 47 years) with a history of hypertension and renal stones

George Redpath is a former sheep farmer from Australia and has now settled in the UK. He is obese (BMI 33.9 kg/m^2) and has a history of hyperuricaemia. He has a small kidney stone and is being treated with allopurinol. The consultant wants his diet reviewed in terms of the risk of both stones and hypertension. His blood pressure is currently 195/100 mmHg. The client is sedentary and was a heavy drinker.

	Day 1	**Day 2**
Breakfast	2 rolls filled with bacon Doughnut Mug of tea with whole milk	2 rolls filled with bacon Cherry muffin Mug of tea with whole milk
am	Mug of tea Cheese scone with butter	Mug of tea Slice of white bread with garlic sausage
Lunch	Leftover Chinese duck dish (from the night before) with pancakes Lemon chicken (box from supermarket) Glass of cola lemonade 2 plums 1 cream cake Mug of tea	2 sesame bagels 6 slices of peppered German sausage Glass of chocolate milk 1 apple turnover Mug of tea
pm	2 glasses of lager (with friend)	Prawn sandwich on brown bread Mug of tea
Evening meal **(19.15 hr)**	Minced meat pie (serving to serve two) with pastry top and bottom Large serving chips Peas and carrots 6 oz chocolate bar	Glass of chocolate milk Large sirloin steak (10 oz) Large serving potato wedges Glass of lager Serving sticky toffee pudding Mug of tea
Supper	2 glasses of lemonade 4 crackers, two large lumps of cheddar cheese	Frozen cream-filled pastry thing Mug of tea

Questions to consider

(1) Inspect the diary entries and comment on the likely overall health risk, with particular respect to hypertension.

(2) Explain how the diet could be re-structured both qualitatively and quantitatively to improve Mr Redpath's health.

(3) What might be the particular dietary and lifestyle priorities for this client?

(4) Assuming that the 'new' diet might be modified to reduce risk of future uric acid stones, what may be the approach to take, and why?

(5) Explain the nature and weight of evidence implicating diet with the development of renal stones and comment briefly on what best practice might be in terms of general approaches to management of the client.

Diary 7 Reactive hypoglycaemia

The diary of a young woman (aged 36 years) with a history of light-headedness

The patient describes episodes of shakiness, dizziness and irritability which resolve on eating. She has to carry food everywhere with her and snacks frequently. She is 5 ft 2 in and weighs 7 stone and is otherwise healthy. She is keen to consult a dietitian and the general practitioner asks her to keep a diary and symptom record prior to a therapeutic consultation. She lives alone and has tried to cut out pasta and bread. She is a keen canoeist (weekends) and cycles to work.

	Day 1	Day 2
7 am	*Cup of fruit tea* *Glass of high energy glucose-based drink*	*[Feeling really hungry]* *2 cups of milky coffee with milk and sugar*
8 am	*Large mug of sweetened latte with a chocolate chip muffin*	*[Feeling shaky]* *Small bowl of muesli-type cereal with whole milk and sugar*
10 am	*[Feeling shaky]* *Piece of sultana bread spread with butter* *Banana* *1 glass of water*	*[Still feeling shaky and perspiring]* *Small chocolate bar* *Glass of high energy glucose-based drink*
12.15 am	*White baguette filled with egg mayonnaise and tomato* *Pot of fruit yoghurt* *Fruit smoothie*	*[Feeling light-headed]* *Avocado, bacon and spinach sandwich (wholegrain bread) tart* *Large glass of fruit smoothie*
1.15 pm	*[Feeling tired, wasted and no energy]* *Glass of water*	*[Feeling light-headed and weepy]* *Couple of squares of chocolate*
7.30 pm **(evening meal)**	*[Feeling hungry]* *Plain boiled pasta with fresh salmon in a cream cheese sauce*	*Tiger prawn, scallop and beansprout stir-fry with noodles* *Glass of low alcohol beer*
10.30 pm **(supper)**	*[Feeling hungry]* *Large mug of hot milk*	*[Feeling hungry]* *Hot-dog, with tomato ketchup in a bread roll*

Diaries

Questions to consider

(1) Inspect the diary entries and comment on the macronutrient composition of the intake, and begin to connect the reported symptoms with the dietary pattern.

(2) Assuming these two excerpts from a seven-day diary are typical of her intake, discuss your findings with a view to formulating appropriate dietary advice for the client.

(3) Put together an action plan for the client taking into account that she reports bursts of activity, such as canoeing for six hours and cycling 28 km.

(4) Prioritise the dietary instructions and explain the key dietary changes (together with mechanisms) that may reduce the risk of hypoglycaemia.

Diary 8 Bowel habit, dietary influences

The diary of woman (aged 60 years) with a history of episodes of diarrhoea

The consultant gastroenterologist has asked for a review of this patient. Her weight pattern coincides roughly with periods of diarrhoea and normal bowel habit. The patient has tried a number of dietary solutions and regularly uses the Internet to search for yet another diet with which to experiment. She is convinced that something in her diet triggers the diarrhoea. She has not eaten bread for years and she is trying to adhere to a dairy-free dietary outline. The consultant is concerned that she may be trying to control too many aspects of her diet to the detriment of her general health. She submits four weeks of dietary records. The following snapshot of her dietary intake is typical.

	Day 1	Day 2
8.30 am	Porridge made with water, sprinkled with sunflower, pumpkin and sesame seeds, served with soya milk Cup of tea with soya milk	Porridge made with water, sprinkled with sunflower, pumpkin and sesame seeds drizzled with honey Cup of tea with soya milk
10 am	Cup of tea with soya milk	Cup of apple and cinnamon tea
1 pm	1 slice of rye bread with soya cream cheese, avocado and tomato Banana	2 gluten-free crackers spread with vegetable pâté and topped with 2 anchovy fillets
3 pm	Cup of tea with soya milk	Cup of peppermint tea

Diaries

	Day 1	**Day 2**
6 pm	6 green olives Glass of white wine spritzer	Handful of gluten-free pretzels Gin and slimline tonic
7:30 pm (evening meal)	Reduced fat houmous with Matzos and various crudités to dip Small portion of vegetable lasagne topped with soya milk/soya cheese Salad vegetables – spinach leaves, tomato, cucumber and celery Cup of tea with soya milk	Small portion of hot smoked salmon in a soya cream sauce with broccoli and leeks Plain boiled corn pasta tossed with some melted soya cheese 2 dried apricots served with small soya yoghurt Cup of tea with soya milk
9 pm (supper)	Glass of water Small handful of grapes	Half a glass of slimline tonic 2 satsumas

Questions to consider

(1) Inspect the diary entries and comment on the broad composition of the intake.
(2) What assumptions may be made about the quality of the entries and attempt to classify the eating pattern of the client.
(3) A number of observations can be made about the food, drink and ingredient selection. Comment fully on what you think is governing food and drink choices.
(4) Assuming that the two days illustrated are typical of the intake, comment fully on the likely intake of macronutrients and begin to make the connection between food intake and weight maintenance.
(5) Discuss and explain the likely approaches taken at the first consultation.
(6) Draw up short- and longer-term nutritional goals for the client.
(7) Discuss follow-up arrangements that may assist in achieving nutritional goals.

Study questions

(1) Explain any nutrition or health implications that may be posed in the diet of a non-meat eater.
(2) Discuss possible strategies that might assist in influencing appropriate food and drink selection in a restrained eater, especially where there is no real clinical evidence for reducing dietary exposure to a particular range of foods (e.g. dairy-free and wheat-free dietary regimens).
(3) Assess the likely wheat and dairy load of your own intake and attempt to classify this as low, medium or high, using a model of healthy eating as your benchmark. What does this tell you about your intake in terms of these food groups?

Diaries

Diary 9 Constipation, hunger

The diary of a young man (aged 28 years) with a life-long history of constipation

Peter Fedora has a desk job, but is an enthusiastic amateur footballer. He is constantly hungry, and his father has heard him prowling about at night looking for food in cupboards and the refrigerator. He is troubled with constipation and is asked to keep a diet diary. He passes two or three small, hard, dry stools (described as sheep pellet-like) every other day. He is keen to resolve his constipation as it is beginning to affect his free time. His weight is stable and his BMI is in the upper range of normal.

	Day 1	Day 2
Breakfast	Rice Krispies, semi-skimmed milk Wholemeal toast and butter Cup of tea, with milk and sugar	Cornflakes with semi-skimmed milk Half bagel with butter Glass of diluting orange juice
am	Cheese scone and butter	Half bagel with cream cheese Cup of coffee (vending machine)
Lunch	Cheese sandwich (white bread)	Tuna mayonnaise on ciabatta
pm	Potato crisps	Cheese snack biscuits
Evening meal (7 pm)	Spaghetti carbonara (bacon and cream) Chocolate mousse 2 chocolate biscuits 1 low alcohol lager	Ham and pineapple pizza (thin 8") Serving baked beans Individual apple pie Custard
Supper (9.30 pm)	Vodka, lemonade and lime Packet of potato crisps	2 'lite' beers Packet of pork scratchings
3 am	Half pint semi-skimmed milk 3 blueberry muffins	Can of cola 4 slices salami

Questions to consider

(1) Inspect the diary entries and comment on the balance and likely dietary exposure to agents implicated in the aetiology of constipation.

(2) Comment on the likely accuracy of the diary entries as may be judged by his weight stable classification.

(3) Glance at the intakes again and assess (using your working knowledge only) intake of NSP, energy and fluid and compare this to target recommendations for intakes of these.

(4) Explain the short- and longer-term nutritional goals for this client with respect to general health and tackling the problem of constipation.

(5)   Taking the diary entries as your baseline or starting point, explain how the client may be advised to move towards a more appropriate diet. Prioritise the changes and draw up a plan over a specific time period.

(6)   What lifestyle changes might assist the client in developing better bowel health?

Diary 10 Obesity

The diary of a young woman (aged 36 years) with a history of obesity

This woman is a little perplexed. She claims to eat 'next to nothing all day', yet still her weight is climbing. She is a psychology graduate but has given up full-time employment (a desk job) to look after her autistic son (Sam, now aged 4 years who has physical, as well as learning disabilities). Her Dad was an Olympic swimmer and her husband is a tri-athlete. She is currently 16 stone 3 lb and of average height. She has a negative body image and is used to large portions of food, no doubt because of previous experiences with a high protein, low carbohydrate reducing diet. She is a keen skier, and goes on a winter holiday every year with friends. She wants to attain her 'wedding weight' of 12 stone 3 lb. You ask her to keep diaries for 4 days; she does so for 14 days. Extracts are given below of both food and drink information together with rough energy expenditure information.

Saturday (home)	Sunday (home)
10.30 am *Bowl of Weetabix with full fat mug of tea* *[Cycled 3 miles, 20 minutes]*	**8.30 am** *1 large double chocolate chip muffin* *1 mug coffee with full fat milk and 2 teaspoons sugar*
1 pm *Baked potato with chicken, bacon, sweetcorn and chive mayonnaise* *Glass mineral water* *Cup of tea* *Fruit scone with butter* *[Cycled 3 miles, 40 minutes]*	**12.30 am** *1 brown bread sandwich, with prawn mayonnaise filling* *Glass of diet lemonade* *[Manual labour, working on decking the patio 60 minutes]*
4.30 pm *Mug of tea*	**6.30 pm** *Bowl of chunky rice and turkey casserole with sweetcorn, carrots and green beans* *Glass of diet lemonade* *Chocolate bar with cream filling*
8 pm *10 home-made turkey pieces in breadcrumbs (deep fried) with garlic mayonnaise* *3 new potatoes* *Portion of cauliflower cheese* *3 glasses red wine* *1 portion apple pie with sweetened double cream*	**7.30 pm** *Banana* *[Drove to see Mum, 60 minutes]* *Bottle of lime and cranberry drink* **10.30 pm** *Cup of tea*

Diaries

Monday (working day)	Tuesday (working day)
8.15 am	*[Cleaned house for 45 minutes, period started today]*
1 large double chocolate chip muffin	
1 mug hot chocolate with cream	**10.30 am**
[Day of meetings]	*1 orange*
	500 ml mineral water
3 pm	*Mango and raspberry smoothie drink*
Large carton pineapple juice	*[Busy and stressful day]*
250 ml mineral water	
High fibre, chocolate chip cereal bar	**2.30 pm**
Packet of cheesy waffle snacks	*1 large fillet haddock (in breadcrumbs, deep fried)*
[Intended to go for swim with husband, but too tired – rested in chair instead]	*Fried egg noodles, ratatouille and hot sauce*
	Handful black grapes
6 pm	*Glass tap water*
[Worked on family tree]	
2 slices brown toast, olive oil spread	**4 pm**
Baked beans sprinkled with cheddar cheese	*Slice ginger cake*
Cup of tea	*Mug of coffee with full fat milk*
2 chocolate cream Easter eggs	*1 glass wine*
[A very stressful day with Sam, it took 2 hr to get him to bed]	*4 squares chocolate*
2 glasses red wine	**9.30 pm**
Handful of Doritos, salsa and chive dips	*[Ate late, Sam playing up]*
Grated, melted Leerdammer cheese	*1 large gammon steak, fried*
	2 fried eggs
	Baked beans
	Glass of orange squash
	3 pancakes with banana and sugar
	Mug coffee

Questions to consider

(1) Inspect the diaries and criticise the extent to which the client's claims and actual intake match.

(2) Comment fully on the content and quality of her typical intake.

(3) Explain how the client might reconstruct her dietary intake in line with healthy recommendations and weight management.

(4) Prioritise the client's short-term nutritional goals.

(5) Based on the energy-deficit model, calculate the client's prescription for energy intake to induce weight loss, and incorporate this into dietary advice information.

(6) Account for the likely second or review consultation, including strategies to promote weight maintenance (as opposed to weight loss).

The referrals
(and contexts)

Referral 1 Letter

Mrs Brown

Study context: referral of client to lower serum cholesterol levels

---

Dear Dietitian

Mrs Brown, 16 Main Street, Horden, Weston-super-Mare
DoB: 04/04/52

I will be grateful if you could see Mrs Brown. She has a
minor coronary atheroma and is an otherwise healthy lady.
She was running a total cholesterol level of 3.8 mmol/l
with an LDL cholesterol level of 2.3 mmol/l. I increased
her atorvastatin to 40 mg/d from 20 mg/d to try to get her
cholesterol down aggressively to lower lipid levels. She
is very keen to have a dietetic assessment. I will be
grateful for your expert advice and assessment of Mrs
Brown.

Consultant Cardiologist

Questions to consider

(1) List the significant points made in the letter, and explain why these are
relevant to the case.
(2) Assuming you see the client, what might be the principal diet and lifestyle changes that may assist in the client's clinical improvement?
(3) Prioritise, with justification, the diet and lifestyle changes suggested in
Question (2) to lead to optimal clinical outcome.
(4) What additional information might you look for in the patient's notes
that may assist you with the consultation?
(5) Mrs Brown is a check-in counter assistant at the local airport. Assuming
the client was responsive and the therapeutic interview went according
to plan, draft a typical letter to the consultant that may be written following the consultation.

Study questions

(1) What is the current clinical target or outcome in a client managing serum cholesterol concentration? Discuss the evidence underpinning the value and note the guideline.

(2) Consider the lifestyle changes that may be appropriate for this case. With which of these might a client find more or less difficult to comply?

Referral 2 Letter

Ms Philpott

Study context: referral of client with irritable bowel syndrome

Dear Dietitian

Ms Fiona Philpott, 23 Andover Rise, Milton Keynes

I would be grateful for your help with this pleasant 23-year-old young woman who has irritable bowel syndrome. Her symptoms first arose in July 2006 when she was on a field trip with her geography class to Russia and had a bad episode of gastroenteritis. Since then her symptoms have continued. She has been seen by a gastroenterologist and a specialist in infectious diseases who have both ruled out inflammatory bowel disease.

We have tried various medications to quell her symptoms but so far, nothing has worked. We are currently trying amitriptyline. I wonder whether she might benefit from some dietary manipulation?

Consultant Physician

Questions to consider

(1) Read the letter of referral and note the major information that might be useful to remember before seeing this client.

(2) The letter typically might contain more information to help guide you through a consultation with the client. Identify, and explain, what additional information might be helpful in this case.

(3) Imagine you see the client and the major dietary 'fault' is that she is a finicky eater and consumes most of her intake after 21.00 hr (60% of her energy intake). She eats relatively well, and healthily, and the meal patterning is:
- Breakfast – nil
- Lunch – two apples and a low fat yoghurt
- Evening meal – a large meal, containing large servings of lean meat/fish with pasta or potatoes, followed by some form of fruit dessert
- Supper – crackers and cheese, and two glasses of red wine while marking in front of the television

Document these findings in her notes.

Study question

(1) What might the major clinical outcomes be for such a client and discuss the contribution that may be made by diet and lifestyle intervention.

Referral 3 Letter

Mrs Young

Study context: referral of client with obesity and other dietary restrictions

Dear Dietitian

Mrs Polly Young, 14 Moorpark, Pontypridd

I will be grateful if you could see this 31-year-old woman who is keen to lose weight and receive some general advice about eating healthily. She is on lithium and phenelzine for depression, and finds dietary restrictions with phenelzine quite difficult to follow. She reports that certain foods cause bloating.

General Practitioner

Questions to consider

(1) Indicate the main features of the referral that may guide the dietitian in making preliminary judgements in planning a first consultation.

(2) Outline the dietary priorities likely to unfold as the consultation proceeds, in terms of both weight management and possible dietary causes of bloating.

(3) Consider the impact of likely compliance issues presented by the various medications prescribed for the client.

(4) The client weighs 85 kg (height 1.60 m). Calculate the energy requirements likely to induce modest and regular weight loss.

(5) Formulate a plan of dietary intervention for the client and indicate how this may change over time as the client loses weight.

Study questions

(1) Research the foods/food agents known to be implicated in the development of symptoms of bloating. What is the weight of evidence for each of the foods included in your findings?

(2) The elements of dietary intervention in clients with bloating might include both reducing severity of symptoms and preventing of symptoms. Discuss strategies to assist both.

Referral 4 Letter

Mrs Leadbetter

Study context: referral of client with iron deficiency anaemia and coeliac disease

Dear Dietitian

Mrs Marion Leadbetter, 17 Cherry Tree Lane, Cirencester

This intelligent young woman has had irritable bowel syndrome for about 12 years and is chronically tired with profound evidence of iron deficiency anaemia. Blood work and duodenal biopsies confirm the diagnosis of coeliac disease and I have given her the address of Coeliac UK. I understand she has been manipulating her diet with the help of the Internet. I will be grateful if she could have a sound education on how to reduce her exposure to dietary gluten and I would value your expert input here.

Consultant Gastroenterologist

Questions to consider

(1) Inspect the referral letter and identify the main indicators that may guide a first therapeutic interview with the client.

(2) Comment fully on the nutritional and dietary priorities for the short- and longer-term of such a client and construct a likely consultation checklist to act as a framework for the interview.

(3) Comment on use of the Internet to inform dietary guidance in patients with coeliac disease.

(4) Comment on the role of Coeliac UK in the management of clients with this condition.

(5) What monitoring and follow-up arrangements would you recommend and why?

Study questions

(1) What may be the longer-term implications of non-compliance with a gluten exclusion diet?

(2) How might dietary adherence be encouraged?

(3) Comment fully on the emphasis you would give to reinforce good intake of calcium and give reasons why.

(4) Evidence suggests some patients in this client group may be lost to follow-up. Comment on the purpose of adequate follow-up arrangements.

Referral 5 Letter

Mr Grant

Study context: referral of client with hypothyroidism and related obesity

Dear Dietitian

Mr George Grant, 14 Old Course Road, St Andrews, Fife

I would be grateful if you would see this delightful fellow, who is originally from South Africa. He has had recent problems with periodic hypokalaemic paralysis and Graves's disease. His thyroid function has been difficult to control; he is currently on 25 micrograms thyroxine and 20mg carbimazole daily and remains euthyroid. His weight is causing him undue angst (108.8kg) which is not helped

by having two young children around with all the trappings
of their diet. He has trouble exercising due to an old
hip complaint. Thank you for seeing him.

Consultant Physician

Questions to consider

(1) Inspect the referral letter and indicate the information that may help
govern a possible therapeutic interview.
(2) Identify the drugs mentioned, and indicate their principal modes of
action.
(3) Explain the main diet and lifestyle strategies for this client that will assist
in weight loss in the short term and weight maintenance in the longer
term.
(4) Discuss fully the evidence that is supportive of the role of physical activity in obese and overweight subjects.

Study questions

(1) Explain the role of thyroid function in achieving and maintaining normal
body weight and discuss the disordered pathology resulting in hypothyroidism and weight gain.
(2) Discuss the possible resistance to weight maintenance and management in clients with hypothyroidism.
(3) Devise possible strategies to assist with weight management in this
group of patients.

Referral 6 Letter

Ms Horvig

Study context: referral of client with abdominal pain for elimination diet

Dear Dietitian

Ms Ester Horvig, The Manse, Shotton, Tyne and Wear

I would be grateful for your help with this pleasant 30-
year-old IT specialist originally from northern Finland.
She has been living in the UK for some 12 years. She has

been experiencing difficulties for the past 18 months with
abdominal pain, bloating and painful defecation that
appears to be associated with certain foods and relieved
by fasting and colonic irrigation.

I have done a formal food allergy screen and have found
no evidence of coeliac disease or common food intolerance.
I would be pleased if you would see Ms Horvig with a
view to establishing an elimination diet. I have no doubt
that she will be able to send you a diet diary
electronically!

Consultant Gastroenterologist

Questions to consider

(1) Inspect the referral letter and formulate an opinion of the major avenues
of investigation that may be worth pursuing in preparation for a first
consultation with this client.
(2) Explain the possible associations between the client's abdominal symptomatology and dietary intake.
(3) Diagnosis of common food allergic disease has been discounted by the
physician in favour of an elimination diet. Discuss the principles of a full
elimination diet and indicate the compliance issues for the client.
(4) Which dietary agents may be implicated in, or attributed to, the development of the symptoms described? What bearing will this have on any
exploration of diet as a likely cause of symptoms?

Study questions

(1) Explain the level and nature of information required to be documented
by the client and discuss interpretation of results during and following
the implementation of a full elimination diet.
(2) Comment on the current medical thinking in the use of an elimination
diet in the determination of food allergic disease.

Referral 7 Nutritional screening

Mr Al-Khatim, Room 221

Study context: referral of client following radical prostatectomy and prophylactic
chemotherapy

The following extract (nutritional screening information) is slipped under your office door. Note the checks (✓) to indicate level of risk for each of the categories contained within the information. The patient is four days post-surgery and is soon to start chemotherapy. He has a nutrition-risk score of 6, indicating LOW nutritional risk.

Referral

Weight loss in last three months (unintentional)
No weight loss   ✓
0–3 kg
3–6 kg
>6 kg

Body mass index (kg/m^2)
20 or more   ✓
18 or 19
15–17
<15

Appetite
Good appetite, manages most of three meals
Poor appetite, poor dietary intake – eating less than
    half meals provided   ✓
Appetite virtually nil, unable to eat, NBM for more than
    four meals

Ability to eat or retain food
No difficulties eating, able to eat independently, no
    diarrhoea or vomiting   ✓
Problems handling food (dependent eater), may have diar-
    rhoea or vomiting
Difficulty in swallowing: needing modified consistency,
    problems with chewing, slow to feed, with diarrhoea
    and vomiting   ✓
Unable to take food orally or voluntarily, unable to
    swallow, severe diarrhoea and vomiting, malabsorption

Stress factor
No stress factor
Mild minor surgery, minor infection
Moderate chronic disease, major surgery, infections,
    fractures, pressure sores
Severe multiple injuries or fractures, burn injury, deep
    pressure sores, sepsis, carcinoma/ malignant
    disease   ✓

Questions to consider

(1) Examine the five categories in the screening information that will assist in the identification of nutritional risk. Indicate how each may have a contribution in affecting the client's nutritional risk.
(2) The screening tool indicates the level of risk currently experienced by the patient. Assuming that you will see the patient following receipt of screening information, identify the likely processes and procedures undertaken by the dietitian prior to seeing the client.
(3) You see the client. What might be the appropriate approach to take, and what information would you give the patient?
(4) What practical measures are likely to be commenced to meet nutritional requirements?
(5) What monitoring procedures would you establish and why?

Study questions

(1) Make the distinction between nutritional risk and nutritional status and indicate clearly what the purpose of a screening tool is.
(2) How often should the nutritional risk assessment be completed and why?

Referral 8 Nutritional screening

Mrs Collins, Room 401

Study context: referral of client following anterior resection of bowel (cancer of colon)

The following extract (nutritional screening information) is sent to you by internal hospital mail. Note the checks (✓) to indicate level of risk for each of the categories contained within the information. The patient has a relatively poor prognosis and is currently being investigated for metastases. She is three days post-operative. The nutrition score is 13, representing HIGH nutritional risk.

```
Weight loss in last three months (unintentional)
  No weight loss
  0–3 kg
  3–6 kg      ✓
  >6 kg
```

Body mass index (kg/m^2)
  20 or more
  18 or 19   ✓
  15–17
  <15

Appetite
  Good appetite, manages most of three meals
  Poor appetite, poor dietary intake – eating less than
    half meals provided   ✓
  Appetite virtually nil, unable to eat, NBM for more than
    four meals

Ability to eat or retain food
  No difficulties eating, able to eat independently, no
    diarrhoea or vomiting
  Problems handling food (dependent eater), may have diar-
    rhoea or vomiting
  Difficulty in swallowing: needing modified consistency,
    problems with chewing, slow to feed, with diarrhoea
    and vomiting   ✓
  Unable to take food orally or voluntarily, unable to
    swallow, severe diarrhoea and vomiting, malabsorption

Stress factor
  No stress factor
  Mild minor surgery, minor infection
  Moderate chronic disease, major surgery, infections,
    fractures, pressure sores
  Severe multiple injuries or fractures, burn injury, deep
    pressure sores, sepsis, carcinoma/ malignant
    disease   ✓

Referral

Questions to consider

(1) Examine the five categories in the screening information that will assist in the identification of nutritional risk. Indicate how each may have a contribution in affecting the client's nutritional risk.

(2) The screening tool indicates the level of risk currently experienced by the patient. Given the information contained within the tool, indicate the likely priorities for nutritional care, and why.

(3) You decide to see the client. What might be the appropriate approach to take, and what information would you give the patient?

(4) What practical measures are likely to be implemented in order to meet nutritional requirements?

(5) What monitoring procedures would you establish and why?

Study questions

(1) Explore the literature indicating the evidence for the use of nutritional screening tools. Give a commentary on how sensitive they might be in determining nutritional risk.

(2) Explain the concept of the nutritional screening tool to a nurse who asks you to do so.

Referral 9 Nutritional screening

Mr Roundman, Room 613

Study context: referral of a diabetic client following de-sloughing of big toes (gangrene)

The following extract (nutritional screening information) is sent to you by internal hospital mail. Note the checks (✓) to indicate level of risk for each of the categories contained within the information. The patient has a poor understanding of the importance of diet. He is obese and has diabetes and was admitted with gangrene of his big toes (BMI 36 kg/m^2). The nutrition score is 4, representing LOW nutritional risk.

Referral

```
Weight loss in last three months (unintentional)
  No weight loss
  0-3 kg      ✓
  3-6 kg
  >6 kg

Body mass index (kg/m²)
  20 or more    ✓
  18 or 19
  15-17
  <15

Appetite
  Good appetite, manages most of three meals    ✓
  Poor appetite, poor dietary intake - eating less than
    half meals provided
  Appetite virtually nil, unable to eat, NBM for more than
    four meals
```

Ability to eat or retain food

No difficulties eating, able to eat independently, no diarrhoea or vomiting ✓

Problems handling food (dependent eater), may have diarrhoea or vomiting

Difficulty in swallowing: needing modified consistency, problems with chewing, slow to feed, with diarrhoea and vomiting

Unable to take food orally or voluntarily, unable to swallow, severe diarrhoea and vomiting, malabsorption

Stress factor

No stress factor

Mild minor surgery, minor infection

Moderate chronic disease, major surgery, infections, fractures, pressure sores ✓

Severe multiple injuries or fractures, burn injury, deep pressure sores, sepsis, carcinoma/ malignant disease

Questions to consider

(1) Examine the five categories in the screening information that will assist in the identification of nutritional risk. Indicate how each may have a contribution (or otherwise) in affecting the client's nutritional risk.

(2) The screening tool indicates the level of risk currently experienced by the patient. Given the information contained within the tool, indicate the likely priorities for nutritional care, and why.

(3) You decide to see the client. What might be the appropriate approach to take, and what information would you give the patient?

(4) The patient is to be discharged. What dietary priorities are there for the client and discuss how these may be communicated to the patient and his wife.

(5) How might the client be followed up and why?

Study questions

(1) The use of nutritional screening may be described as essentially for the malnourished client groups. Discuss the application of these tools, and the interpretation of clinical information for an obese client, as in this case.

(2) The client has avoided contact with the diabetic clinic for about 15 years. Assuming you find the client a little reluctant to comply with dietary instruction, create a virtual entry for the client's case notes using suitable notation convention.

Referral 10 Handwritten note

Mrs Lundquist, Room 408

Study context: referral of a diabetic client with gestational diabetes with limited information

You find the following note placed on your desk and you note that the patient is due for discharge the same afternoon.

We have a Mrs Lundquist here – in for some routine tests – she needs to see a dietitian before going home. Can you see her today before 3 pm?

Student nurse (Ward 10 – Gynae)

Questions to consider

(1) Comment fully on the means of communication and route of referral (referring agent) in terms of ethics and usual hospital protocol.

(2) After numerous telephone calls, you discover the potential client has gestational diabetes. What additional information would you want to ascertain, and why?

(3) Assuming you have the time to see the client, explain the processes that might assist you in determining how important it is for you to see her.

(4) Explain the possible areas of dietary intervention that may be appropriate for the client.

(5) How might the client be followed up, and why?

The mini-cases
(and contexts)

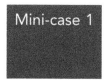

Desmond Paul is a 30-year-old web designer with multiple sclerosis. He spends most of his time in a wheelchair but is not confined to one. He is referred for slow but steady weight loss (BMI 28 kg/m^2). Assessment of height and weight using equipment are not possible.

Question to consider

Discuss the methods open to you to assess his nutritional requirements with a view to establishing appropriate dietary habits.

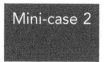

Moira Raymond is on a nasogastric feed to improve her nutritional status following major gastrointestinal surgery (anterior resection). The surgeon insists that her feed should be continuous, with no rest periods.

Question to consider

Put forward a case for 'resting the gut' during a bolus feeding regimen and discuss how you might try to persuade the consultant about the evidence that resting the gut is good practice.

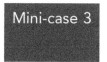

Amy Williams is a successful businesswoman who is referred to the dietitian. Although she is happy with her business life, she is unhappy about her lack of control when it comes to managing her weight. She refuses to be weighed.

Question to consider

Discuss how assessment of this client might proceed, as a prelude to dietary intervention.

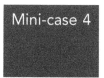

Nutritional screening largely centres on identification of nutritional risk in the malnourished population. An unconscious obese (BMI 35 kg/m^2) man is referred from the accident and emergency department following a fight and has multiple fractures to his ribs and upper body.

Question to consider

Explain what special considerations might be invoked for this obese client through the process of nutritional screening and determination of his nutritional requirements.

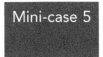

Alex Smith is a busy salesman who was diagnosed as having coeliac disease about a year ago. He declined the invitation to be referred to the dietitian, instead deciding to pick up dietary information, as necessary, from the Internet.

Question to consider

Discuss any compliance issues that may result from obtaining dietary information in this way, and from bypassing the therapeutic interview with a dietitian.

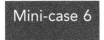

Djan Aziz is a young man in his twenties and has type 2 diabetes. The doctor suspects non-compliance with his medication(s) and his diet.

Question to consider

Explore the issue of non-compliance in this Asian client and discuss how you might motivate the client to adhere to his diet.

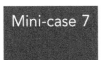

Rebecca Milne is a 21-year-old girl who plans to get married in about six months time. She self-refers to the dietitian and is keen to lose 10 kg so that she can fit into the wedding dress she purchased during the winter sales.

Question to consider

Consider the issue of aggressive weight loss both in the short and longer term in the context of health risk and management issues.

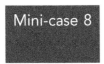

Mabel Smith is 78 years of age and recently widowed. She falls whilst planting spring bulbs and has undergone a unilateral hip replacement. She experiences post-operative sepsis. She has a BMI of 19.1 kg/m^2.

Question to consider

Compare and contrast nutritional priorities and how nutritional requirements may be met during the six-week post-operative stay in hospital and during the rehabilitation period following discharge.

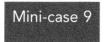

Sam Horner is a professional rugby player and was carried off the field unconscious following an over-enthusiastic kick by an opponent.

Question to consider

If the patient remains unconscious for a period of one week, discuss the possible feeding strategies available to feed the prop forward.

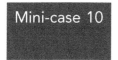

Noel Pearson is a second world war veteran (pilot) who has undergone a recent radical prostatectomy with prophylactic radiation. He has lost 8.2 kg in the immediate three-month post-operative period.

Question to consider

Assuming the weight loss is exacerbated by the radiotherapy, explain the nutritional approaches that may assist in stemming further weight loss.

Mini-cases

The commentaries

The commentaries: the cases

Consideration of the cases reveals the following observations. They may help inform appropriate dietary, nutritional and lifestyle approaches and advice.

Case 1

- Initial impressions of the case indicate that the client is an older person and probably has long-standing diabetes. She is taking metformin, suggesting that she may be overweight. There are lifestyle considerations: her alcohol consumption may exceed recommendations and she is a heavy smoker. Her physical activity may be moderate to high depending on how involved she is with managing the market garden. Her diet is likely to be fairly healthy with emphasis on fresh foods and may be the reason for her complaining about the hospital food. Her pre-operative weight is not given and should be ascertained for monitoring purposes. Hospital dosage of metformin is two tablets each day, suggesting the client over-medicates for whatever reason. A complaining patient may need careful handling.
- Assessment should involve checking all usual diabetic parameters to have some baseline information for future comparison. This must include weight (and weight history), dietary intake information and estimation of the HbA$_{1c}$ level. A full dietary history of recent intake is crucial (it is likely that access to diabetic care services has been poor) together with an historical account of diet (to note changes over time). An account of medication history will also be useful in planning care. Lifestyle assessment will provide valuable information (alcohol consumption, smoking habits and physical activity judgment).
- Short-term goals include establishing a healthy diet (based on a lower fat/starchy carbohydrate intake) with regular meals and snacks to meet broad nutritional requirements and encourage achievement of normal/ideal weight (to assist glycaemic control). Inspection of current diet will reveal how far the client is from a Mediterranean-style intake. Recent weight loss may not be a worry (surgical trauma) in an otherwise healthy patient, assuming spontaneous appetite returns after surgery (she is complaining and so is likely to be hungry from the information given). High blood sugar following surgery is not unusual, but the dose of metformin may need to be kept under review, as also the need to consider combination treatment, such as metformin with acarbose or insulin, to improve glycaemic control temporarily.
- Longer-term goals include achieving ideal weight targets, maintaining a regular intake of starchy carbohydrate, sustaining appropriate lifestyle changes (including a check of alcohol consumption and smoking habit) and reviewing use of anti-diabetic medication. Consideration of smoking cessation may be a priority.

Commentaries

- Monitoring should include assessment of all significant diabetic parameters and follow-up arrangements planned according to access to care. It may be appropriate to manage the patient from the UK and arrange annual review at a convenient diabetic centre.
- Handling of a complaining patient will require tact and diplomacy but may offer another opportunity to further discuss aspects of care, including use of diabetic products. Recommendations for use of products specifically formulated for people with diabetes should follow advice as documented in clinical guidelines (Diabetes UK).

Case 2

- Initial impressions of the case indicate that the client has end-stage renal failure (urea and creatinine levels); the degree of hyperphosphataemia is expected with his level of renal function. The potassium concentration is within the normal range, but the patient may not be eating well. Concentrations of sodium are low; this may be due to fluid overload. The patient is short of breath, secondary to fluid overload and anaemia.
- Priorities for medical intervention include treatment of anaemia and blood pressure, together with arranging access for dialysis and initiation of phosphate binders (and possible vitamin D therapy).
- Priorities for nutritional intervention include investigation of appetite and dietary intake. Assessment of whether the patient is meeting nutritional requirements for energy and protein is important. The patient should be encouraged to reduce the level of salt intake to a 'NAS' diet. Dietary phosphate intake should be assessed, but it may not be appropriate to give advice about reducing exposure to dietary phosphorus as appetite may be poor.
- The patient needs to meet nutritional requirements, and requirements for protein, energy and major nutrients should be calculated according to clinical guidelines: energy: $(11.9 \times 67) + 700 = 1497\,kcal/d + 25\%$ (stress factor) $= 1869\,kcal/d$; protein: $1.2 \times 67 = 80\,g/d$. Sodium intake: $80-100\,mmol/d$. Phosphate intake: $0.55\,mmol/kg/d = 37\,mmol/d$. Potassium intake: $<1\,mmol/kg$.
- Advice to the patient should attempt to align the intake with requirements and reinforcement of protein and energy intake seen as a priority. The patient should be given advice about how to manage salt restriction and fluid intake. The intake of high potassium foods should be checked and curtailed as appropriate. Advice about dietary phosphate restriction and use of phosphate binders may be given at a later stage.
- In the longer term, a history of weight, appetite and symptoms (nausea, vomiting and bowel function) may be useful. A regular diet history will help prioritise the main areas for dietetic intervention (likely to be salt, fluid and nutritional support). The rationale for dietary changes, together with the aims of intervention, should be discussed with the patient and appropriate literature provided.

Commentaries

■ The difficulties presented by the case may centre on language barriers and the problem of providing advice that is understood; presence of the patient's cousin or an interpreter will be helpful. Possible financial difficulties (unemployment) are likely to impact on dietary intake. The patient is also a heavy smoker; smoking cessation should be considered.

Case 3

■ Initial impressions strongly suggest that the patient is in end-stage renal failure (increased concentrations of urea and creatinine). Increased concentrations of alkaline phosphatase and phosphate are consistent with renal bone disease, a consequence of end-stage renal failure. The alkaline phosphatase and phosphate concentrations warrant further investigation and treatment. In addition, blood calcium should be investigated (is likely to be low) and levels of parathyroid hormone should be assessed to check progress and severity of renal bone disease. Treatment may include alfacalcidol and phosphate binders together with dialysis and dietary intervention.

■ Requirements for major nutrients should be calculated: energy: 25 kcal/kg (accounting for PD fluid) = 1663 kcal/d together with increased requirements in peritonitis (BMR + 10% stress factor). Protein: 1.2 g/kg IBW = 80 g/d, increased in PD to 1.3–1.5 g/kg = 86–9 g/d. Fluid requirements should be addressed (ultrafiltration on PD) together with account of energy absorption from indwelling dialysate.

■ In the longer term, blood investigations should be done routinely, clinical chemistry regularly assessed and any necessary interventions planned as appropriate. Monitoring of dry weight is important.

Case 4

■ The client presents as an intelligent, older man who has presumably kept quite well until this recent period of illness. It may be useful to ascertain fluid status to determine if this may influence clinical chemistry values. It would be useful, for example, to know what the patient's urine output is. The patient is probably quite well nourished, given the concentration of albumin; other parameters may suggest a good dietary intake (e.g. level of phosphate).

■ Many of the clinical parameters are consistent with a decline in renal function (levels of creatinine, urea, phosphate and potassium). The level of haemoglobin is very low, and the patient is clinically anaemic. The serum/plasma concentration of both potassium and phosphate is above the clinical cut-off level, and reducing exposure to dietary phosphate and potassium will inform clinical goals. If the patient is taking ACE inhibitors or is a diabetic, then potassium levels may be higher than expected. This should be checked.

Commentaries

■ Short-term goals include improving the patient's nutritional status and reducing symptoms (by medical and dietary means) to enhance the patient's feeling of well-being/quality of life. The patient's diet should be aligned with recommended intakes of protein (to manage elevation of urea level) and energy (to manage elevation of creatinine level) to move the patient nearer to optimal nutritional status. Since intakes are set according to dry weight, it is important to ascertain how much of the 96 kg is wet weight. The patient is also clinically obese and therefore energy requirements may be set at the lower end of a range. An energy intake of 35 kcal/kg/d and a protein intake of 0.6–0.7 g/kg/d conforms with dietary/clinical guidelines (assuming a dry weight of 90 kg, energy requirements may be 3150 kcal/d and protein requirements may be 54–63 g/d). It may be appropriate to set the energy intake at about 2500 kcal/d and monitor clinical chemistry/weight parameters. It may be prudent to limit the patient's dietary phosphorus intake (to 30 mmol/d, assuming the patient is not malnourished) by avoiding phosphate-rich foods, and limit dietary potassium intake (to 1 mmol/kg/d) by avoiding intake of potassium-rich foods (e.g. swapping potatoes for pasta and rice) and by not using quick cooking methods (e.g. steaming and microwaving). The patient should be established on a NAS diet (80–100 mmol/d), and treated medically for anaemia. It will be important to establish the concept of a small portions approach to implement the modest protein restriction. Vitamin and mineral supplementation should be given routinely according to hospital policy.

■ In the longer term, the key approach will be to monitor the patient to avoid malnutrition, and this will involve strict and frequent monitoring of dietary compliance. It may be useful to check arm anthropometric measurements, clinical chemistry and dietary intake (dietary history) and adjust aspects of the diet accordingly. Appetite will improve as a result of reducing the concentration of urea and resolution of anaemia; there may be a risk of breaking the diet if the appetite is unchecked (use of phosphate binders may be useful). Longer-term dietary measures should include lipid-lowering advice and ensuring as healthy an intake as the level of dietary restriction permits. Protein intakes should be monitored closely to ensure an intake of predominantly HBV protein. Renal function should be kept under review and relevant medical interventions implemented as necessary (e.g. use of phosphate binders).

■ The patient's care may revert to the USA, and the treatment plan should be communicated to the patient's home care unit/facility.

Case 5

■ The case presents as a slightly underweight (BMI 18.8 kg/m²) older woman who may be at risk from malnutrition. Her social situation may not be ideal (isolation and limited access to food). There is a need to know the magnitude of recent weight loss.

■ It is important to check that the patient is adequately hydrated, as this may alter interpretation of clinical parameters. The dietary intake may be poor (concentration of albumin); other parameters are indicative of diminishing renal function and some data suggest longer-standing renal insufficiency and a level of bone involvement (low concentration of calcium and raised concentration of phosphate). It will be useful to know whether the patient is anaemic (and treat this medically). Bicarbonate levels are lower than the reference standard, but medical intervention is not usually required until the critical values of <10 mmol/l or >40 mmol/l are reached. Assessment of dietary intake is important, to act as a base-line for both interpretation of clinical data and to inform potential dietary intervention.

■ The primary short-term goal is to avoid malnutrition and ensure that the patient has reasonable access to food and drink to encourage her to meet nutritional requirements. Energy requirements, based on actual body weight, suggest an intake of 1523 kcal/d (35×43.5). Clearly, there is a need to know how much weight the patient has lost, which will assist in formulation of the energy prescription. One of the goals may be to improve weight status, in which case requirements need to be adjusted upwards. It may therefore be appropriate to plan an intake based on achieving normal BMI, and therefore, an ideal weight (say 50 kg). BMR $= (10.5 \times 50) + 596 = 1121$ kcal, together with a PAL factor (light activity) of $1.56 = 1749$ kcal/d. Protein intake, based on an intake of 0.6–0.7 g/kg/d (clinical guidelines), would indicate an intake of 26.1–30.5/d. This may not be sufficient to support the goal of achieving optimal nutritional status. There may be a need to improve protein intake to make good the loss of LBM and intake may be increased to patient tolerance (with monitoring of parameters). The prescription for intake of energy and protein may be approximately 1800 kcal/d and 50 g protein/d, respectively.

■ Concentrations of potassium and phosphate require to be monitored; there may be no immediate need to implement restriction of dietary intake for either of the nutrients as both components are just outside the reference ranges. If restriction is implemented, it will not be aggressive and will involve modest restriction (watching intake of rich sources).

■ In the longer term, the client should be encouraged to follow as healthy a diet as the level of restrictions permit, although it is important to feed, rather than to restrict, to ensure the patient does not become malnour-ished. Compliance with achieving energy and protein intake and ulti-mately achieving a normal BMI will be goals, in the context of a practical (NAS) diet. Periodic dietary inspection will be useful together with weight monitoring. Arm anthropometry may not be prudent with an older client, but routine clinical chemistry may reveal changes in status that require intervention. Memory assessment may be useful in determining likely future adherence with dietary intake.

■ Clearly there are issues with whether the patient can comply with dietary instructions when discharged, and monitoring may be possible through community arrangements. If the patient is not managing to consume

Commentaries

ordinary diet, then perhaps the use of a nutritional supplement may be worth considering. One sip feed daily may be useful, although will depend on whether fluid restrictions are in place (500 ml plus the previous 24 hr output). Nutritious snack foods may be worth promoting. There may be a tendency to purchase convenience or ready-to-serve meals. These will be sodium-rich and the patient should be encouraged to eat more fresh foods; this is dependent upon her limited income (she is also feeding a family cat).

Case 6

■ Initial observations suggest that it may be unrealistic for the client to achieve a 'healthy' BMI. He should first concentrate on the shorter-term goal of achieving 10% of initial or baseline weight. It may be useful to consider the cause of gluttony. He is relatively inactive.

■ Assessment: since it may be unreasonable to expect achievement of 'normal' BMI, a decision needs to be made about what may be reasonable and achievable. He is single and therefore consideration may be given to the nature of support (family and friends) available between review appointments. It may be useful to find out why he is no longer a professional cricketer (personal choice, his weight or injury) as this may affect motivation. Exploration of the self-confession of gluttony may be useful.

■ Short-term goals may be influenced by the need to modify eating behaviour: what is the cause of gluttony? (For example, it may be comfort eating.) He also needs to be advised about watching so much television. It may be helpful to explore whether the greater energy demands of his professional cricketing days have been sustained into his non-playing periods, and whether his physical activity levels have fallen. It will be useful to reduce serving sizes and increase physical activity as his injuries permit. The client needs to be motivated to change behaviour resulting in inappropriate eating. The intake should be balanced.

■ In the longer term, goals will be to encourage adherence to portion-control measures, to ensure healthy eating and to further increase physical activity. Approaches should ensure behavioural change, with goal setting and rewards. The use of food diaries may be considered to engage the client with his management.

■ Dietary intervention may be planned using the appropriate predictive equations (BMR) and guidance on calculating physical activity levels: BMR = (15.1 × 155) + 692 = 3032.5 kcal; PAL = 3032 × 1.5 = 4548.75 kcal (1.5 = light occupational activity and moderate non-occupational activity). To assist weight reduction, the intake may be planned around a deficit of 1000 kcal = 3500 kcal/d. NICE guidelines should be consulted and a motivational interviewing approach used.

■ With morbid obesity, regular weight checks may be considered (four weekly). Waist circumference measurement may be useful and total body fat monitoring used if equipment is available. Dietary advice regarding healthy eating should be given at the commencement of treatment and the client encouraged to complete a seven-day diet diary prior to review appointments.

Case 7

- Initial observations suggest that the current usual diet may be affecting clinical chemistry and that the client is maintaining weight outside the optimal range (65–81 kg). The client's lifestyle and lack of physical activity may be contributing to his weight; his alcohol consumption is not specified.
- The offshore diet will contribute significantly to outcome, due to the time periods involved. The diet will contribute to all factors raised in the blood profile. The client's weight is stable, so the current diet and lifestyle factors need to contribute to a shift towards negative energy balance. There may be a need to consider the offshore catering arrangements to provide healthier options (if not already doing so); it will be important to ascertain whether it is the client's food choice or the provider's meals that are inappropriate. The client may be encouraged to drink more fluids.
- Short-term nutritional goals could be to establish a routine pattern of three meals a day, as opposed to the current erratic pattern. Priority may be given to reducing the portion size of the lunch and providing a healthy eating option at the evening meal. An increase in fluid intake ($35\,ml \times 93 = 3255\,ml/d$) should be reinforced. The client should be encouraged to consume less protein and aim for two main servings only per day.
- Dietary intervention may be planned using the predictive equation for energy based on BMR and PAL: BMR = $(11.5 \times 93) + 873 = 1942\,kcal$; PAL = $1942 \times 1.4 = 2718\,kcal$. To achieve weight loss, the intake may be planned around a deficit of $500\,kcal = 2200\,kcal/d$. NICE guidelines should be consulted and motivational interviewing approach used.
- Longer-term goals could include increasing physical activity, reducing intake of puddings and increasing uptake of healthier options. The client will benefit from reducing the quantity of spreading fat and should be encouraged to use a lower fat option within the context of healthy eating dietary advice (including aspects such as dairy foods and sodium/salt content of diet).
- The client may be reviewed at clinic when onshore, and probably every 4–6 weeks. Weight should be checked, together with repeat blood work and 24-hr urine investigations. The completion of a food diary prior to appointments may be helpful. It may be useful to request a menu from the rig and make some suggestions for improvement or use it to assist in informing the client's choice. It may also be useful to explore access to a gym or facilities either offshore or onshore.

Commentaries

Case 8

- It may be expected that this patient will experience a significant decrease in appetite and intake in the first few days post-operatively. Creation of a J-pouch is a relatively new surgical procedure and there are no long-term follow-up studies as yet. The surgery is often accompanied by an ileostomy, which may be reversed after about eight weeks to allow the pouch to heal.
- In the short term, nutritional requirements post-surgery will increase, mainly due to wound healing. The colon is the site of water absorption, so an increase in fluid requirements is likely and may initially be met with intra-venous hydration. It is good practice to give advice on increasing fluid intake. Fluid status (intake and output) is also usually monitored and the colour of urine noted. Small frequent meals may prevent excessive pressure on the pouch. Avoiding foods that may be indigestible and risk causing obstruction (whole nuts, sweetcorn and seeds) of the pouch output may be useful. Avoidance of hot and spicy foods is advisable to prevent burning sensation in the peri-anal region. Food avoidance should be individually tailored. There is an increased requirement for intake of calcium and patients with ulcerative colitis maintained on steroids may be advised to take 1500 mg/d, to reduce risk of developing osteoporosis. The use of supplements may reduce effort of the diet to supply all this.
- In the longer term, goals include reaching an acceptable weight (from the low BMI baseline). Some kick boxers may wish to aim for a specific weight category. This can be discussed with the patient. It may be prudent to reduce strenuous exercise activity in the immediate post-operative period and resume later, depending on recovery.
- Monitoring will include weight parameters, satisfactory resolution of anaemia and adherence to a reasonably healthy diet to meet weight goals.

Case 9

- A detailed dietary history (possibly a food diary) will provide useful information especially about intake of NSPs, fat and sugar content of the diet together with establishing a picture about alcohol consumption, fluid intake and meal patterning. It will be useful to check whether the client has experimented with diet in the past and what success this has yielded. This information may inform core dietary advice (e.g. perceptions of dietary triggers of symptoms). An account of bowel habit may form a useful baseline against which the impact of any future dietary change (diarrhoea versus constipation) can be assessed. Encouraging the client to report weight changes over time and the presence of other symptoms may be informative (headache, fatigue).
- Initial advice will be informed by findings (above) and needs to address the erratic meal patterns and excessive coffee consumption, together

with increasing intake of appropriate fluids. If dietary intake of fat and sugar is high, then advice should be given to bring intakes into line with healthy recommendations. Bloating may be alleviated by gradually reducing intake of dietary fibre (initially) for a trial period of no longer than four weeks. The client may need the support of a bulking agent during this period. Advice on increasing energy expenditure will be helpful. The client should be reviewed (at four weeks). A key point will be to establish regular eating.

■ If symptoms improve, the content of dietary fibre should be gradually re-introduced until the optimum level is reached (ideally as high as possible without exacerbating symptoms of bloating). The desired clinical outcome will be to establish the patient on a healthy eating, balanced diet with regular and frequent food intake.

■ If there is no improvement in symptoms, then a trial of an exclusion diet (for two weeks) may be useful, as well as reducing dietary exposure to reported and perceived problem foods, such as wheat, milk and dairy products, eggs, chocolate, caffeine and alcohol. The patient should self-monitor by keeping a food diary and symptom record and this should be reviewed at the end of the trial period. If there is no improvement in symptoms, then the plan should be to revert to a healthy eating approach. If the patient experiences symptomatic improvement, then advice about gradual re-introduction of foods will be required and an individualised diet planned, based on simple exclusion of trigger foods. Regular dietary review may be important here to ensure a nutritionally balanced intake.

Case 10

■ Initial impressions of the case indicate a woman who may enjoy a comfortable lifestyle (trip to the Philippines) and is therefore likely to consume a diet exceeding nutritional requirements. Although she does not exercise, she has a job in which she has to stand. She is showing signs of the consequences of obesity (shortness of breath and back pain) which may be motivational issues to be considered at a consultation. Dieting history appears to have had poor outcome (suggesting compliance issues) but may be a useful discussion point. She has had access to slimming pills, which may suggest yet another motivational issue. The GP is reluctant to prescribe further supplies, which suggests she is not likely to meet prescribing criteria (client should demonstrate modest weight loss prior to consideration for prescription). The case therefore presents major motivational issues, requiring the use of motivational counselling and CBT.

■ Assessment should centre on dietary intake, and a full diet history or seven-day diet diary may be useful to ascertain intake of macro-nutrients and eating behaviours. A lifestyle assessment may be useful, although clues suggest poor exercise behaviour (poor mobility).

■ Short-term goals include reducing health risk by encouraging the client to consume a healthy diet, based on a model of a lower fat, high intake

Commentaries

of starchy carbohydrate foods (perhaps based on the BoGH), and engaging in regular weight-bearing exercise on days not at work. The intake may be planned on the energy-deficit principle, thus energy requirements need to be calculated. Assuming she is of average height (170 cm), then with a BMI of 36 kg/m², her actual weight is about 104 kg. Her energy prescription can be calculated: BMR = (8.7 × 104) + 829 kcal = 1734 kcal; in addition, to include physical activity, PAL = 1.56 (light activity) × 1734 = 2705 kcal and incorporation of an energy deficit of 5–700 kcal = total daily energy prescription to induce weight loss = 2200–400 kcal/d.

■ In the longer term, goals include achieving negotiated dietary changes (stepwise) and targets for weight, which are likely to be small steps towards eventually achieving good clinical outcome. Follow-up arrangements to monitor parameters should be negotiated with the client and may be monthly, eight weekly or six weekly, when weight loss begins to progress so that support can continue. The GP should be kept informed of progress, as there may be a wish to consider the client for pharmacological treatment at some point when appropriate weight loss has been demonstrated for prescribing purposes.

Case 11

■ The client presents as an older woman who blames her weight issues on her thyroid problem. However, she is euthyroid with use of drugs, and therefore her thyroid function should not affect her likelihood to gain weight. Blaming thyroid function, or prescribed thyroid medication, may be the client's way of explaining weight gain, and will certainly be a discussion point for the initial consultation. The client is beginning to show effects of obesity (back pain) which may be motivational. Weight history shows success, due to both dietary and pharmacological intervention. A high fat/high protein diet has induced short-term weight loss but this could not be sustained. Clients following diets in which protein and fat are allowed 'ad libitum' usually have issues related to portion control, and eat large quantities of these foods. A consultation will want to capitalise on the success of trying to lose weight in the past and the potential of future dietary intervention to do the same. The use of pharmacological agents may suggest further motivational issues (low self-esteem, and possibly financial issues).

■ Assessment should centre on dietary intake, and a full diet history or seven-day diet diary may be useful to ascertain intake of macro-nutrients and eating behaviours. A lifestyle assessment may be useful to plan physical activity or other appropriate intervention.

■ Short-term goals include reducing health risk by encouraging the client to consume a healthy diet, based on a model of a lower fat, starchy carbohydrate intake (perhaps based on the BoGH), and engaging in regular, modest weight-bearing exercise. The intake may be planned on the energy-deficit principle, thus energy requirements need to be calculated. Assuming she is of average height (165 cm), then with a BMI of 35 kg/m^2, her actual weight is about 94 kg. Her energy prescription can be calculated: BMR = $(10.5 \times 94) + 596$ kcal = 1583 kcal; in addition, to include physical activity, PAL = 1.3 (inactive) $\times$ 1583 = 2058 kcal and incorporation of an energy deficit of 5–700 kcal = total daily energy prescription to induce weight loss of 1500 kcal/d. The diet should be planned for a client managing on limited means; the dietary instruction should be centred on CBT and delivered with motivational counselling techniques. Particular attention should be given to managing portion control, especially of protein-containing foods.

■ In the longer term, goals include achieving negotiated dietary changes (stepwise) and targets for weight, which are likely to be small steps towards eventually achieving good weight outcome. Follow-up arrangements to monitor parameters should be negotiated with the client and may be monthly, eight weekly or six weekly, when weight loss begins to progress, so that support can continue. The GP should be kept informed of progress. Community support classes may be a possibility to maintain interest and motivation in aspects of lifestyle, including cooking, fitness, general health issues and weight management.

Case 12

■ Initial management centres on adequate and sustained hydration and encouraging the patient to increase and maintain a sensible fluid intake (at least some of the weight loss will be fluid loss). The use of electrolyte replacement solutions may be beneficial to stem electrolyte losses; intravenous fluids may be indicated.

■ In the longer term, prevention of further weight loss is a clinical goal. This will be achieved by monitoring dietary intake and reviewing weight parameters. The patient may benefit from use of nutritional supplements and this can be assessed at the dietary review. Some solid foods may not be tolerated very well, and will vary from person to person. In extreme cases, and especially where a long period of diarrhoea is expected, a nasogastric feeding regimen may be implemented. Vomiting can be managed by medical means.

■ Maintaining an acceptable weight may require the use of an energy-dense, higher protein intake. This may take several months and will depend on BMI, actual weight loss and weight history. Requirements for protein, energy and fluid should be calculated and adjusted as the patient improves.

Case 13

■ Rose presents as an otherwise healthy, overweight person. She has a BMI of just over 30 kg/m^2, and the question is whether she is stressed due to the presence of *Staph. aureus* (no CRP or WCC values are given)

Commentaries

and if she has lost weight rapidly (due to sepsis). With a BMI of <30 kg/m², she may be fed to meet basal energy requirements only (1469 kcal, approximately 1500 kcal/d). Monitoring must ensure that she is meeting this requirement as a minimum, and also meeting requirements for micronutrients (especially zinc, copper and selenium). She should be given protein to meet 75% of requirement as she has a BMI <30 kg/m², which would be about 75 g/d. Fluid intake and balance should be monitored as the patient may be pyrexial.

■ Following re-admission to hospital, primary treatment objectives are to provide nutrition support to meet nutritional and fluid requirements and to educate her on a suitable diet for hospital and home (when appropriate). She should not consider dieting again until the wound has healed and is infection-free.

■ Low concentrations of haemoglobin will affect wound healing ability and it is important to ensure that protein sources are HBV. Intake of iron-rich foods should be encouraged and consumption of vitamin C should be promoted (to assist with iron absorption). Folate and vitamin B$_{12}$ levels should be checked, and if necessary, monitored. Low blood potassium concentrations should be tackled (encouraging intake of potassium-rich foods), however it is not stated how low these levels are (care needed to avoid cardiac arrhythmia). The cause of hypokalaemia should be ascertained (e.g. blood loss). Potassium levels should be ascertained and monitored as part of ongoing care.

Case 14

■ There is some evidence to suggest that elimination of certain foods from the diet may reduce symptoms (pain and inflammation) in patients with rheumatoid conditions. Gradual re-introduction of foods and the re-emergence of symptoms may result in consideration of these foods being eliminated from the diet on a long-term basis. A case such as this presents difficulty: no single diet will suit all patients as all clients have different needs.

■ There is increasing evidence that the use of omega-3 fatty acids is beneficial. These supplements are known to reduce production of certain substances during the inflammation process. Indeed, trials show that omega-3 fatty acids may be a suitable alternative to use of non-steroidal anti-inflammatory drugs (NSAIDs) in effecting at least partial pain control.

■ Records of food intake (diet diary) may provide useful information on which to base dietary intervention, such as meal times, snacking behaviour (intake in relation to lifestyle), an estimate of energy/fat content of meals and snacks, the variety of foods consumed (or lack of) and the intake of dietary fibre and fluid (the patient complains of constipation). Intake of total (and type) of fat is important: the client has lupus, and has increased risk of hypercholesterolaemia (she should be advised accordingly). Snacks and convenience foods may carry more of the at-risk ingredients: it is therefore important to review intake of these foods (and advise accordingly).

■ Lifestyle issues need to be considered with caution and any advice given should be realistic. There will be poor ability to exercise (due to lupus) and this will therefore limit the ability to lose weight (although weight loss is a priority). Dietary manipulation is likely to be the major strategy in losing weight, and therefore dietary goals need to be realistic in targeting weight loss. Readiness to change behaviour also needs to be assessed; her attitude to weight loss is important (motivation), especially when relying on dietary intervention alone. She does work at home and activity is related to the degree of arthritic pain (she may sit most of the time); she is constipated: dietary advice should centre on trying to alleviate constipation. A family history of cancer of the bowel may be motivational. There is a need to explore why the patient eats so erratically: is this through personal choice, work pattern/social issues or through lack of planning her intake?

■ It is important to base dietary intervention on the common theme of obesity and arthralgia and dietary advice may focus on the BoGH to encourage dietary variety and healthy eating (vitamins and minerals). Omega-3 fatty acid supplements may be a useful addition to the diet, together with promotion of foods known to contain rich amounts of these (e.g. oily fish). This will be especially beneficial due to the high risk of CHD with lupus. An energy-deficit diet will reduce weight and assist with pain control of joints (should be estimated based on BMR and PAL, together with a suitable energy deficit of 5–700 kcal/d). The pattern of regular meals is important. The use of fruit as snack foods is practical and appropriate.

Case 15

■ Initial thoughts about the case indicate that the client is symptomatic, and this may help with motivation and ultimate compliance with dietary guidance. It may be wise for the dietitian to liaise with the organisers of the race concerning food provisions – if they are assuming that participants will use a lot of dried food and highly processed provisions, then this may pose significant problems for a client on a gluten-free diet. In view of the strong family history, the client is probably familiar with the principles and some of the practice of the diet, and may have good ideas about how he will cope with dietary intervention. On the farm, isolation may be the major problem, in terms of what is available locally, and he may need to be encouraged to do a bigger shop in town to stock up on basic food items.

■ Diagnosis has been confirmed, and therefore he needs a gluten-free diet to manage symptoms and reduce longer-term risks (e.g. lymphoma, osteoporosis and anaemia). His social situation (isolation) needs to be worked around, for which he may need support and encouragement.

Commentaries

- Short-term goals include bringing his symptoms under control and sorting out the immediate problems of the ship race.
- In the longer term, goals include managing other races, based on experience with the present one and reducing health risk (e.g. development of osteoporosis). Dietary intervention should conform with clinical guidelines (e.g. British Gastroenterological Society). The steatorrhoea, flat biopsy and strongly positive antibodies should provide the basis and introduction to dietary counselling. If the biopsy was less flat, and diarrhoea less obvious, this would pose motivational issues for the first appointment with the client. Helping him to avoid becoming overweight is a priority and this should be discussed at the outset.
- The intervention would take the form of a gluten-free diet based on healthy eating and with emphasis on an adequate intake of calcium.
- Degree of symptom relief and compliance with the diet would form the basis of monitoring arrangements. Regular long-term follow-ups at fixed intervals should be planned, reducing to annual review as he stabilises and makes all the necessary changes. His hobby is clearly part of his life, but this may conflict with intake of a gluten-free diet.

Case 16

- Initial thoughts about this case include raising awareness with the MDT. If not working as part of an eating disorder team, the dietitian must consider scope of practice and if necessary liaise with other professionals or refer to psychological services. This is a chronic case, and may need a significant period of treatment (16–20 weeks in the first instance). Approaches need plenty of time as the client may have low self-esteem, may have a fear of being judged, may be feeling guilty and may find it difficult to trust a dietitian. There is a history of bulimic eating disorder and there is a risk of relapsing into vomiting cycle, thus prevention is a priority. The presence of depression means that the dietitian must be aware of effects of mood change; the risk of suicide, self-harm or detrimental behavioural change must be communicated to the psychiatrist. BMI classifies the client as obese; this may compromise longer-term health. The client has a part-time job; this is positive as time is occupied and she has a social outlet.
- The diagnosis of bulimic eating disorder/bulimia nervosa necessitates a CBT approach and education and counselling must focus on the damaging effects of the disordered eating. A risk assessment may be completed (the psychiatrist) and a clinical assessment may include investigation of urea, electrolytes and LFTs with haematology. Assessment of the main manifestations is important: binge behaviour, alcohol consumption, obsessive exercising and vomiting behaviour as this will inform the basis of educational and treatment priorities. Also useful to ascertain is whether the client misuses laxatives, diuretics or uses recreational drugs. The client is obese, and therefore weight monitoring should be considered. A discussion of feelings about her size is important, in view of poor

self-esteem and confidence. Assessment of readiness to change behaviour is also important (may be a measure of ability to achieve goals).

■ The initial consultation should take place in a relaxed, controlled and confidential environment. Use of core counselling skills is imperative, including, tact, empathy and congruence in a non-judgmental manner. A history of current symptoms (sore throat, dental erosion, swollen glands, vomiting blood, abdominal pain, dizziness and irregular periods) and binge-cycle development over time will be useful. A dietary history will provide information about triggers for binges. Access to information about social situations may provide clues to issues about home, family, childcare conflict. Knowledge about the involvement of any other services will be useful together with access to support networks (family, friends or professional support workers). Height and BMI may be monitored in a sensitive way. A care plan should be formulated.

■ Short-term goals, centred on education, may aim to relax the grip of the binge/starve cycle. The physiology and biology of appetite and weight control may be used to normalise eating pattern by establishing three balanced meals a day and introducing a light snack to reduce hunger at night (to reduce the risk of night time binges). Stopping binges is a priority, and the aim will be to reduce this in stages if unable to stop outright. Any dietary restrictions during the day should be discouraged as this can trigger binges in the evening. The risks of long-term obesity should be discussed and a realistic target for weight loss agreed (e.g. 0.5–1.0kg/week). Alcohol consumption should be ascertained and brought to sensible limits. A sensible approach to exercise should be encouraged to reduce risk of obsession. The client should be encouraged to keep a food and mood diary to record, and subsequently understand the links between food and drink consumption and emotions. The client should be allowed to explore her thoughts and feelings to help her challenge negative thoughts and develop alternative patterns of thinking that produce positive feelings and behaviours around food and body image.

■ In the longer term, counselling should centre on relapse prevention and reinforce regular eating and development of appropriate responses to hunger and satiety cues. Introduction of low glycaemic index foods may be useful (to assist with regulation of blood sugar and therefore help with satiety). Craving for sweet food may be ameliorated by advocating a 'low calorie' chocolate drink or a serving of fruit. Weight should be monitored regularly (perhaps monthly) and targets for weight loss kept within reasonable limits. The client should be encouraged to enjoy foods within a variety of social settings. Monitoring may also include ongoing food and mood diaries, eating behaviour questionnaires and anxiety and depression scoring.

■ Educational approaches should focus on 'normal': healthy weight, balanced diet and sensible approaches to alcohol consumption and exercise. Complications of bulimic eating disorder may be motivational (osteoporosis, fertility issues, depression and low self-esteem). A healthy eating model of education may be used and may be modified by

Commentaries

priorities (NICE/RCP or other guidelines). Counselling and education should engage with the increasing level of client motivation.

■ The particular challenge presented by this case may be that the client may not be ready to change behaviour. Reducing bingeing symptoms may increase the risk of self-harming and other inappropriate behaviours.

Case 17

■ The case presents the picture of an obese client with a history of raised uric acid levels. The client has been motivated to seek help via the Internet to reduce his risk of stones, but he needs to lose weight and adopt a more scientific approach to manage his risk of developing more stones. He is likely to have a high intake of protein and salt (two factors which assist calcium excretion, and therefore enhance stone-forming risk) together with a high intake of purines (meat). Whilst 80% of stones contain calcium, there is no real evidence that dietary restriction reduces risk of stone development. The effects of dietary intervention on the reduction of the risk of developing are likely to be small, but perhaps worthwhile to consider. The client is likely to be maintained using appropriate drug intervention (allopurinol).

■ Whilst the client may be at cardiovascular risk, initial assessment should concentrate on dietary (diet history or diet diary) and lifestyle (exercise, intake of alcohol and salt) assessment. Weight parameters may be noted with a view to monitoring from baseline and calculation of energy requirements.

■ Short-term goals include implementing dietary changes to reduce the risk of formation of stones and for general health improvement (healthy eating and to encourage weight loss and improve cardiovascular health). Implementation of an energy-deficit intake, based on healthy eating (high in starchy carbohydrate and lower in fat) with particular focus on reducing protein and salt intake will assist in achieving weight loss and reduction in the risk of formation of stones. The dietary intake may be centred on an energy prescription based on: BMR: $(103 \times 11.6) + 879 = 2074$ kcal; in addition to a PAL factor (light activity) $= 2074 \times 1.55 = 3214$ kcal together with an energy deficit of 5–700 kcal $= 2500$–2700 kcal/d. The intake should be planned to include salt restriction (probably to the level of NAS, or 80–100 mmol/d), alcohol restriction to recommended levels and protein modification to about 1 g/kg/d (to reduce exposure to both protein and purines). An emphasis on greater intake of NSPs will be useful (stone formation is less likely with cereal/vegetable-based protein intakes). The client must *not* be encouraged to have oily fish (high in purine content) and should switch to lower fat dairy products. Approaches must focus on reducing portion sizes, especially of protein-containing foods. Fluid intake should be increased to about 2 litres to 3 litres per day to promote production of dilute urine.

■ In the longer term, issues include general health improvement via diet and lifestyle improvement, including engagement in light and sustained physical exercise. Monitoring should include weight parameters and dietary compliance, especially with regard to protein and salt intake. The client may be monitored frequently in the first instance (every 8–10 weeks) and thereafter revert to the care of either a practice nurse or occupational health nurse. Cardiovascular parameters may be worth exploring in the context of general health, with dietary and lifestyle reinforcement as necessary.

Case 18

■ Initial thoughts presented in this case include peer pressure at the photo-agency and perhaps the presence of underlying issues (which may require a team approach). The deliberate intention of not involving family may be counterproductive; family is often integral to therapy, especially in a client so young. The client's life is not stable (living with both families) and there are issues of confidentiality. Dietary restraint is practised and her weight could fall further. Vomiting is associated with health risk (electrolyte disturbance).

■ Assessment may focus on cycle history and cause, anthropometric measurements and medication. Energy requirements may be calculated using predictive equations. It may be useful to discuss family dynamics, especially in relation to not wanting family members to know about the problem. A dietary history, both current and historical may be useful to ascertain eating behaviours in the development of, and during, the eating disorder. A history of alcohol use may provide useful information. Physical parameters may be checked, including blood pressure, cardiovascular monitoring and dental health, and symptoms of sore throat, abdominal discomfort, amenorrhoea, risk of osteoporosis, hair loss, poor skin condition and presence of lanugo hair on arms. Psychological parameters may also be checked including degree of cognitive impairment, presence of anxiety, depression and suicide ideation. Engaging the client with the issues will be important: Does she have insight into the cause? How ready will she be to change behaviour? Is she aware of the risks associated with her behaviour? The dietitian can use these to form the basis of motivational approaches. Confirmation of diagnosis will be important – is it bulimia nervosa or purging-type anorexia nervosa?

■ Short-term goals, centred on education, may aim to engage the client with the binge/starve cycle and the physiology, biology of appetite and weight control to normalise eating pattern by establishing three balanced meals a day and stopping episodes of bingeing. Prevention of further weight loss is a priority together with stabilising weight within healthy limits. A sensible approach to alcohol consumption, exercise patterns and general healthy eating is important. The client will benefit from education regarding the risk of low BMI and malnutrition, with emphasis on lean body mass loss. A food and mood diary will help the client to address issues between food, emotions and triggers (associated with negative thoughts). The client should be allowed to explore thoughts and their influence on her behaviours.

■ In the longer term, goals include reinforcement of good behaviours (healthy eating, regular eating and the development of appropriate responses to hunger/satiety cues). Vomiting and bingeing episodes must stop and the aim is to achieve and maintain a target (and healthy) weight. Sensible approaches to alcohol, drug use, eating and exercise, food and weight control should be reinforced and encouragement given to eating in company especially throughout the day. A motivational approach should be used to provide reassurance and encourage the client to maintain behavioural improvement in stages.

■ Monitoring should include strategy to manage risk of relapse and include regular weight monitoring (perhaps monthly) and targets for weight gain kept within reasonable limits. The client should be encouraged to enjoy foods within a variety of social settings. Monitoring may also include ongoing food and mood diaries, eating behaviour questionnaires, and anxiety and depression scoring.

■ The particular challenge of this case is the reluctance to involve family and may result in the family eventually tackling the problem inappropriately and creating greater conflict.

Case 19

■ Initial thoughts presented in this case include: that polycystic ovarian syndrome may be the cause of the obesity, and not purely because of excessive energy intake or lack of physical activity. There is a need to tackle insulin resistance. A motivational key will be that weight loss improves the hormonal abnormalities and increases the likelihood of ovulation and pregnancy.

■ Polycystic ovarian syndrome is also associated with increased risk of diabetes, raised blood pressure and hypercholesterolaemia due to long-term resistance to insulin, obesity and hormone imbalances. It is important to consider all aspects of diet that may contribute to these factors (healthy eating, physical activity, intake of salt, quality and quantity of fat, weight patterns).

■ It may be important to establish why the client has stopped taking the contraceptive pill and whether she is planning a pregnancy (if so, pre-pregnancy counselling may be considered). Motivational factors include pregnancy planning and increased fertility associated with weight loss. It will be useful to consider goal setting, rewards, use of pharmacological agents (metformin), access to 'exercise on referral schemes' and review of energy requirements to assist with reduction of weight. Height and assessment of physical activity will be required to calculate baseline energy requirements.

■ Energy requirements should be calculated as a basis of a modified energy-deficit eating plan to induce slow and steady weight loss (with goals). The client may be monitored (weight, waist circumference) and goals adjusted as short-term goals are achieved.

Case 20

- This case presents a male patient (probably between 30 and 60 years of age) who has experienced aggressive weight loss (6%) at day 9 post-operatively. Initial thoughts are that the patient needs to meet estimated requirements to maintain weight and for healing of surgical wounds. In addition, control of nausea will be important. The patient is unlikely to meet nutritional requirements on oral diet; establishing a supplementary nasogastric feed to prevent further weight loss will be important.
- Nutritional requirements may be estimated/calculated using standard predicative equations. Energy requirements may be estimated using BMR = $(11.4 \times 76.2) + 870 = 1740$ kcal, together with the addition of 25% (assuming mobile on the ward) and a further 400 kcal (to promote weight gain) = $2200 + 400$ kcal = 2600 kcal/d. Protein requirements may be estimated: 0.17 gN $\times 76.2$ ($\times 6.25$) = 80 g/d. Fluid requirements = 35×76.2 = 2600 ml/d.
- The plan would be to feed 1000 ml high energy feed (1.5 kcal/ml) overnight to provide 1500 kcal, and 60 g protein. Oral diet would supply 700 kcal + 30 g protein. An energy-dense fat emulsion (e.g. Calogen) would supply the additional 400 kcal/d. The patient would need advice on appropriate menu choices to meet the desired energy and protein intake (700 kcal and 30 g protein), and may include selecting good protein and energy sources such as full cream milk, fortified soups and thick and creamy yoghurts and puddings.
- It is important that the patient is monitored throughout all stages of feeding and that care is implemented according to local protocol/referral policy and is adequately documented in medical notes.

Case 21

- Initial impressions indicate that there are cultural issues (is the client Muslim?) and that religious/cultural eating practices may contribute to current symptoms. In addition, young children in the family unit may have an impact on eating habits. Knowledge of traditional foods (Pakistan) and their nutritional profile may assist in guiding dietary advice (the client may be asked to bring empty packets/food containers to appointments).
- Baseline medical assessments appear to be complete and therefore problems may very well be related to a faulty dietary intake.
- Short-term goals may be ascertained by conducting a dietary assessment. The client may also benefit from a discussion about her concerns in relation to medical concerns and with her nutritional status. An exploration of the likely dietary causes of symptoms may investigate the following: intake of dietary fibre (is she meeting the recommendations?); fluid intake (does she meet the requirements?); iron sources (is intake of both haem and non-haem sources adequate?); eating patterns (are these regular?); and exercise (how does this compare with recommendations?) The client would benefit from healthy eating advice with reinforcement

Commentaries

of adequate intakes of fluid and iron in conjunction with regular eating.
- In the longer term, goals may be to achieve and maintain intake of a balanced diet and one that meets micronutrient requirements. Reinforcement of good intake of iron-rich foods together with those foods that enhance iron absorption would be useful. A discussion about soluble and insoluble NSPs would assist in exploring the importance of dietary fibre in context. Continuing advice about the importance of meeting fluid requirements may help (especially in hot weather, illness and during exercise). The client's perception of a low fat diet may help in aligning the diet with a healthy intake. Review appointments may be assisted by completion of a food diary. Fluid requirements should follow sensible advice (35 ml/kg) = about 2000 ml/d.
- The first review appointment may be in four weeks from first encounter, when weight and general progress can be monitored. Bowel habits may be followed up, in light of effects of ferrous sulphate (constipation) on bowel habit. This may be reviewed in favour of a non-constipating iron supplement (Spatone).

Case 22

- The principal difficulties associated with managing this client are her poor short-term memory and limited communication ability.
- Assessment would include nutritional screening on admission, in addition to weight history (could use old medical notes for old weight parameters) and an account of dietary intake (food record charts from hospital; review of current dietary intake from the daughter, nursing staff or perhaps even the staff from the day centre). The daughter would be the main source of information from which to guide management and may include: a weight loss pattern (when did weight loss start? what is the extent of weight loss and what is the client's usual weight?) and an opinion about appetite, and therefore, intake (perhaps taking a full dietary history, to include what and when the client eats, what are her dislikes/likes and preferences?). Other useful information includes an account of her recent appetite, and how this has changed over time, whether the client has chewing or swallowing problems and what kind of textures the client can manage. A report of eating experience at the day centre may be useful together with any other help that is given with meal provision. The extent to which the daughter copes may be worth noting.
- The options for continuing monitoring should be considered, and include weekly weighing, daily food record charts and regular nutritional screening. In the short term, the principal goal will be to enable the client to meet nutritional requirements in the provision of a high protein/energy-dense diet, served as finger-type foods. Arresting weight loss is also a priority. Other important issues include encouraging the intake of sweet foods, such as milky puddings and drinks, and the consumption of forti-

fied foods (such as butter added to potato, milk powder added to milk-based items). The use of supplements may be considered, and any 1.5 kcal/ml milk or juice-based supplement is indicated (perhaps first trying chocolate/milk-based drinks, as client appears to prefer chocolate). The use of a fat emulsion-based supplement (e.g. Calogen) may assist in reducing weight loss; the use of a Procal-type supplement may be added to milky puddings and drinks. Some supplements may not be tolerated and milkshake-style supplements, with added ice cream, may be offered. The use of brightly coloured trays and assistance with eating at meal times may encourage intake.

■ In the longer term, dietary goals include achieving and maintaining good nutritional status together with stemming further weight loss. It is essential that the daughter is able to cope with her mother's diet and some time needs to be spent talking her through practical measures that will enable goals to be met. Liaison with colleagues in the MDT will be important, including the occupational therapist who will be able to assist with specialised cutlery and feeding aids. It is also important to arrange access to support services (e.g. carers, who may be able to help with feeding) and it may be useful to consider additional sessions at the day centre. Discussion with the daughter may include: the main principles of the high protein, energy-dense diet and the judicious use of food fortification. The session may be reinforced with the use of published information (NAGE, Alzheimer's Society) and reference to peer-reviewed websites, which may have links to other websites that assist in locating local help with care. If use of supplements is proving successful, then these may be continued at home, and reviewed by community dietitians.

■ The nutritional care plan will assist in achieving dietary goals; it is important that all members of the care team (including the residential care home) know their role in delivering, at least in part, nutritional goals. Monitoring weight and dietary intake should continue as part of routine observations, and the need for supplements reviewed in light of these observations. The community dietitians may wish to train residential care home staff if training is seen as a need. Care home staff should be encouraged to offer small, frequent meals/snacks to support the diet.

Case 23

■ The case presents as a child failing to meet adequate growth when plotted against 'normal' growth pattern (height, weight or BMI). Poor nutritional intake and sub-optimal nutritional status may be key features in this case.

■ Initial assessment may include checking retrospective growth data from parent-held records or other sources. Poor feeding is likely to result from poor oral co-ordination and poor motor skills, and it will be important to conduct a full assessment including videofluoroscopy by an appropriately skilled SLT. Aspiration may occur, which leads to repeated chest infections and further compromises nutritional status. It is important, therefore, to consider the medical view of the overall clinical condition. The patient needs multi-disciplinary assessment of feeding skills, nutritional status and overall clinical condition, before intervention can be agreed. There is a need to investigate if some of the problems are behavioural, or have underlying clinical causes.

■ Short-term nutritional goals centre on whether the patient is safe to be fed orally for both liquids and solid food. If the patient is deemed safe to swallow, use of nutrient-dense fluids are appropriate (age-appropriate supplements, addition of energy-dense foods to meals, such as butter, margarine, cream, cheese, sugar) and the use of full fat (not low fat) and avoidance of low sugar products. The patient and parent/care-giver requires a full explanation that energy requirements may not be met otherwise and that although this differs from advice given to normal children, it is important to meet requirements for growth. Thickened fluids may be required to prevent aspiration; appropriate advice should be given. If swallow is unsafe for fluids or solids, then discussions with family members is important regarding the more invasive forms of nutrition support, including nasogastric or gastrostomy feeding. This can be devastating for families and requires careful discussion and counselling.

■ Monitoring of uptake of oral diet/feeding regimen and nutritional status is important to ensure requirements are being met. Psychological assessment will be important to assess behaviour and any necessary behavioural interventions implemented. An MDT approach is essential as the aetiology of feeding problems in cerebral palsy is likely to be multi-factorial.

■ Monitoring of height and weight is usually done six monthly on a UK centile chart. A regular and detailed diet diary may check dietary intake. A multi-disciplinary review is important and may include school and other carers.

■ The case presents the potential to easily mistake a behavioural feeding issue which may have an underlying cause as opposed to a nutritional problem. It is therefore important to consider behavioural issues and how meal times can be used to communicate other problems for management.

Case 24

■ Any paediatric dietetic intervention should begin with accurately plotted weight and height data to assess and monitor nutritional status. No data are given, and so the initial thought must be to obtain data and plot on a Down's-specific growth chart. Initial impressions of the case include the need to assist with feeding behaviour, ensure long-term growth is consistent with anticipated norms in Down's syndrome and that the quality of the diet is acceptable. There will be a need to get a detailed history of meal times – who is there, what food is given and how independent is the patient?

■ Assessment of the case indicates that the history points up eating behaviour issues, rather than concerns about nutritional status. Priorities may centre on issues related to hydration, given the details of drooling and mouth breathing. It may be useful to refer for specialist input: the SLT to assess feeding ability, the occupational therapist for advice about use of appropriate feeding utensils, the school and psychologist for social skills assessment and training and the dentist, for assessment of abscesses.

■ Short-term goals include ensuring that the diet and fluid intake is adequate (perhaps from a diet diary) to meet nutritional requirements. If the diet is adequate, then the mother should be reassured. If not, then the mother should be advised of specific concerns and a plan of action negotiated. It may be useful to observe eating during a mealtime to assess eating behaviour. The SLT should review the patient to assess if eating is affected by hypotonia.

■ In the longer term, goals include working jointly with other professionals to improve behaviour at meal times and take advice from the psychologist or school on appropriate methods to improve both eating behaviour and diet quality (e.g. use of rewards, star charts). Immediate changes in dietary intake may not be necessary, since behavioural problems appear to dominate the picture.

■ Monitoring arrangements may include dietary assessment and examining the effect of strategies to reduce parental anxiety around meal times. It is important to include all relevant agencies so that behavioural intervention is consistent.

■ This case is typical of some areas of disability, in that feeding behaviour can be an issue even in the absence of concerns about nutritional status. This can be more difficult to resolve because of the number of people involved (e.g. parents, siblings, grandparents, school staff, respite carers). This may be compounded by the inability to access professionals (e.g. psychologists) who can help the parents achieve sustained behavioural change.

Case 25

■ Initial impressions of the case are that the client is putting her child, husband and hobby (horses) before her own needs, and that her lifestyle needs to be addressed in addition to diet (alcohol consumption and stress). She needs to understand that there is a medical reason for reactive hypoglycaemia, which usually occurs three to five hours after taking food or drink containing glucose (glucose loading).

■ Taking into account the biochemical data, this patient does not have diabetes, but the management may be based on similar principles. Exploration of the events leading up to episodes of reactive hypoglycaemia may be useful in informing the intervention. Using the data provided on her eating pattern, consideration needs to be given to barriers to changing behaviour, such as managing a job, a child and a hobby. The baseline data do not provide all the information required and a full diet history will be required to obtain quantitative data about the diet.

■ Short-term nutritional/lifestyle goals must focus on the patient achieving a regular meal pattern to include starchy, carbohydrate-based foods at every meal. This involves tackling the patient's current perception of starchy foods (i.e. making sure she understands that they are low in energy and why the body needs them as the main source of energy). The rationale behind tackling the meal pattern and inclusion of starchy foods is based on providing the body with a regular supply of carbohydrate to stabilise blood glucose levels throughout the day. The evidence base for this is apparent in published clinical guidelines for diabetes (e.g. Diabetes UK). It will also be important to tackle the issue of the patient's sweet tooth because excessive intake of energy from sweet foods is likely to increase fat as well as sugar intake, and at the same time compromise intake of slow-release carbohydrates and foods with a high vitamin and mineral content.

■ In the longer term, the patient needs help to juggle her home and work life around prioritising her own dietary needs. Helping the patient stabilise weight in the longer term may be useful, instead of watching her weight when competition time approaches. Healthy eating approaches over long, rather than the shorter-term, is the best sustainable approach.

■ The management plan is best communicated in a dietetic consultation based around verbal and written dietary advice, presented in a motivational way, and using counselling skills (reflective listening). Tools such as the BoGH would be an excellent guide to inform healthy eating principles. Any personal targets can be built into the instruction and will be informed by the dietary history. The shift towards achieving the targets set out in healthy eating advice must be gradual and individual aspects of the diet changed in negotiation with the patient. Over time, the changes will build into a consistent and permanent change to dietary habits, especially if the symptomatology is improved (motivational).

■ Monitoring and evaluation (diet history and anthropometry, together with symptom review) should be done at the follow-up clinic, and targets re-negotiated. Compliance issues should be followed up during the consultation period, as the patient may struggle to adhere to the new diet. Social issues may also hamper compliance (family life and work pressure).

■ The case presents several challenges including the existence of barriers to change and embedded beliefs about the nutritional value of starchy foods. The patient does not have diabetes, where the evidence base is strong; the evidence base for management of reactive hypoglycaemia is weaker.

Case 26

■ Before proceeding with consultation and advice, a formal diagnosis of diabetes is required. It is not clear what the diagnosis on board was based on (it could have been based on fasting blood sugar, oral glucose tolerance, or more likely on a finger-prick blood glucose test). There are weight management issues in this case, and possibly other lifestyle factors, such as lack of physical activity. A low carbohydrate regimen/intake based on carbohydrate exchanges is not appropriate for the initial management of type 2 diabetes.

■ Short-term goals include establishing the client on regular meals based on starchy carbohydrate; this involves a movement away from carbohydrate restriction towards a carbohydrate-based diet. The principles of healthy eating should be the approach to take with this client to assist with glycaemic control and health improvement (e.g. increasing fruit and vegetable intake and including oily fish in the diet).

■ In the longer term, goals should address the problem of weight management – this may be achieved with an investigation of portion sizes, activity level and underlying psychological issues influencing dietary intake. Achieving consistent long-term glycaemic control is another principal aim.

■ Implementation of appropriate diet and lifestyle improvement should consider a number of staged interventions, including stepwise approach to dietary change in line with recommendations from Diabetes UK, as the current diet may be a long way from the recommended diet. Small changes, implemented over a long period of time, are required to reduce the risk of non-compliance. The intervention would be based on healthy eating principles, using verbal and written advice and employing CBT techniques (such as self-monitoring and diary keeping). Diabetes UK advocates carbohydrate inclusion at every meal rather than restriction.

■ The patient should be monitored and reviewed at clinic (at 12 weeks initially, and then reverting to six monthly and annual review appointments). A variety of assessments are usual, including diet history, anthropometry (BMI and waist circumference) and a review of targets. Waist circumference is a useful tool to assess cardiovascular risk. Changes in glycaemic control (e.g. HbA_{1c}) can be reviewed at dietetic review. Review dates should be set and depend on progress towards targets and motivation to change (should be assessed initially). There may be many compliance issues in this case (e.g. cultural issues, family influence and the extent to which the patient has accepted the diagnosis of diabetes).

■ Particular challenges presented in this case include overcoming potential barriers to changing dietary behaviour, handling the conflict of information presented initially (on board) and subsequently. The contradictory dietary advice needs to be explored fully at clinic and the advantages and disadvantages of the former and latter diet discussed in the context of the evidence supporting the change. Using a motivational style and a mix of communication skills will enhance transmission of these messages.

Case 27

■ Initial thoughts about this case suggest that a diagnosis of irritable bowel syndrome is likely, although consideration of undiagnosed coeliac disease may be possible (masked by symptoms of irritable bowel syndrome). No information on a weight history is given, nor about the client's attitude to her weight. Is the 24-hr diary typical of the client's intake across a week? The history suggests a poor intake of starchy carbohydrate and a high intake of energy from alcohol. She appears to smoke cigarettes in place of food. There are strong lifestyle influences affecting intake, such as eating out, the timing of meals and the real lack of time to plan and accommodate her intake.

■ Lifestyle issues are possible barriers to changing dietary habits (sugar, alcohol and caffeine consumption) and emphasis should be given to the benefits of changing her diet, such as decreasing bloating risk and encouraging better bowel habit (more regular and more formed stools passed with greater control and less urgency).

■ Short-term priorities include decreasing caffeine intake (incrementally to prevent withdrawal symptoms) and increasing non-caffeine-containing fluids to compensate for diarrhoeal fluid losses and climate (Costa Blanca). Dietary fibre should be increased incrementally with emphasis on soluble-rich sources and including insoluble forms with examples from local cuisine (e.g. pulses and fruit). The introduction of a breakfast would be wise together with encouraging engagement in relaxation (e.g. yoga) and more time for herself.

■ In the longer term, the client should engage with local initiatives for smoking cessation and decrease alcohol to recommended limits. It may be helpful to have some discussion about the feasibility and likely compliance of a wheat-free and/or milk-free diet, or a few foods exclusion diet. The client should be alerted to any local/national irritable bowel syndrome networks.

■ Modification to diet and lifestyle should be monitored; reinforcement of significant issues may occur at review. Psychological support may be useful. Diet may be assessed using a seven-day food and symptom diary, and if feasible, to include a holiday period. Telephone contact may be useful at four weeks and follow-up will depend on local policy.

Case 28

■ Initial thoughts about the case are that the symptoms are typical of an infection and that the CD4 count of <200 makes the patient more susceptible to infections.

■ Baseline information of diarrhoea, fever and night sweats indicates the need to increase fluid requirements; dry rough mouth is characteristic of dehydration and infections mean a heightened inflammatory response.

■ Short-term goals are guided by the possibility of clinical malnourishment (7% weight loss over four weeks) and the need for nutritional support. Hydration is a priority together with salt replacement in view of the diarrhoea (electrolyte replacement therapy). Antiemetic medication may assist with the nausea and nutritional supplements should commence in view of nutritional status. The selection of supplement will be determined by tolerance and diarrhoea. If the diarrhoea worsens, there is a need to consider a semi-elemental sip feed. Depending on the tolerance to oral diet and fluids, the patient may need to be considered for nasogastric tube feeding.

■ In the longer term, goals include aiming for the patient to reach a BMI within the normal range, by supporting usual diet with nutritional supplements, food fortification and food enrichment. The patient requires appropriate dietary advice to include ideas of how to support the diet (above) and a discussion about food safety and basic hygiene may be useful. Dietary issues associated with the exact anti-retroviral agent used will be necessary (started because of the low CD4 count). There may be a need to advise the client to stop running and any general high impact exercising until medically stable and good nutritional status is reached (may be motivational). In view of the immunosuppression, it may be advisable to discontinue any herbal supplementation.

■ Correction of malnutrition may assist in ameliorating the symptoms. Their appearance/disappearance can be reviewed. Progress can be monitored on admission (daily stool charting, food records, biochemistry and general observations such as temperature and blood pressure) and moving towards weekly weight checking. On discharge, there is a need to arrange a prescription for supplements and this should be reviewed in four weeks.

■ The case presents the challenge of whether to commence a full protein or a semi-elemental feed given the presence of diarrhoea. It is also difficult to assess whether there is true malabsorption. Resolution of symptoms will depend on whether the patient is fed nasogastrically. It is usual to establish the feeding regimen and monitor in the first 24 hours and then reassess its suitability.

Case 29

■ The client appears to be motivated, in that he has approached the dietitian, and is therefore accepting that his diet and lifestyle may be improved to influence health risk. His motivation is probably enhanced by his brother's death, but this may only be short lived. He needs to focus on the wider picture of health and into the longer term, rather than concentrating on a quick fix approach.

■ The client's BMI indicates that he is at high health risk; his waist circumference would no doubt suggest the same. Both parameters would have increased significantly from his playing days. His lipid profile is raised, perhaps as a result of a high saturated fat intake, but a closer look at dietary intake in respect of LDL, HDL and triglyceride profile is warranted. A high protein/high alcohol intake combined with possible calcium deficiency and lack of exercise may be influencing bone density parameters.

■ Short-term nutritional and lifestyle goals must centre on reducing the intake of red meat, perhaps cutting this down to one medium, or two small portions a day. Cooking methods may be reviewed, and meat consumed should be lean, unprocessed (contains less salt) and not have added fat in the form of gravy or sauces. Meat should be wet cooked (unlikely, given the specific case), roasted or 'dry' fried, and never fried. Consideration needs to be given to his alcohol consumption, and reducing this if necessary, to target recommendations. The client should be encouraged to undertake regular cardiovascular exercise; a discussion of fitness levels, during and post-rugby playing days may be useful. A healthy eating model of intervention is appropriate, with accent on improving NSP intake, moderation of intake of meat and confining his diet to fresh foods and regular eating.

■ In the longer term, goals must centre on keeping the client engaged with continuing the intervention and making his diet more varied, perhaps with the inclusion of more vegetable, fruit, pasta and fish dishes. Perhaps he could develop an interest in fishing, alongside his hunting abilities? The client has a good appetite and may benefit from hearty food choices such as casseroles, soups and pulses in addition to meat ingredients. Practical and achievable dietary goals should be the approach.

■ A healthy eating model of intervention is appropriate, with particular attention given to portion control (especially of meat). A suitable energy-deficit, healthy eating diet plan may be constructed using predictive formulae: BMR: $(11.6 \times 120) + 879 = 2271$ kcal/d; PAL: $1.55 \times 2271 = 3520$ kcal/d, including a deficit of 5–700 kcal = 2800–3000 kcal/d. This will need to be monitored over time, to readjust the energy deficit in order to maintain weight loss.

■ Monitoring at review appointments (negotiated, but say every 12 weeks in the first treatment year) may check weight and waist circumference. Medical monitoring may check lipid profile and blood pressure. The client's general practitioner may wish to be kept informed of progress towards achieving a healthier lifestyle and dietary intake.

Case 30

■ Initial thoughts may centre on key points: a young woman with breast cancer suggests genetic risk factors and poor calcium status may be due to dietary restraint (does she avoid dairy products?).

■ Initial assessment may consider: patient's age and possible impact of bone density reduction on future quality of life, ethnic origin/lifestyle and the possibility of recurrence of breast cancer. Anthropometric data and history may be useful when planning intervention, to include weight, BMI and weight alterations post-treatment.

■ Short-term nutritional/dietary and lifestyle goals may include: maintaining and improving dietary calcium intake, reviewing dietary intake of vitamin D and maintaining optimal age-specific nutritional status.

■ In the longer term, goals may be to maintain optimal dietary calcium/vitamin D intake, maintain optimal nutritional status and continue (but keep under review) with appropriate calcium supplement.

- Nutritional judgements may be based on a 7-day dietary history (ideally a diet diary/weighed record) and a full computerised nutritional analysis of the intake. Suitable and practical alterations in intake can be planned, based on the analysis.
- An intake of about double the reference daily amount for calcium will reduce rate of bone loss.
- Follow-up arrangements may be planned and dietary assessment repeated and compared with baseline; findings may be documented and the multi-professional team aware of evidence-based interventions specific to the case.
- Care may be required in handling a very young patient with such sinister diagnoses. Interventions should be client focused.

Case 31

- Assessment of the client's dietary intake should ideally take the form of a three-day food diary but compliance is likely to be poor given her social circumstances; a detailed dietary history may be the only option. Initial thoughts of the case are that there is a need for the patient's diagnosis to be confirmed (salicylate sensitivity) as the diet is very restrictive. Salicylates are present in many cosmetic products, therefore a discussion around use of these products is essential (e.g. shampoo, face creams). Use of aspirin and aspirin-containing medications must be assessed. Diet inspection should yield significant information, including types of foods and drinks eaten/drunk, quantity or volume and frequency.
- Dietary advice and information may take the following emphasis: avoid sauces (salicylates are present in many spices) and ready-made foods (e.g. ready-made meals, jar sauces), avoid consumption of wine and spirits, avoid contact with salicylate-containing foods as a topical skin reaction is possible and avoid possible cross-contamination by using separate utensils/chopping boards. Dietary advice may separate foods/drinks into those permitted (i.e. are salicylate-free) and those not permitted (i.e. those containing salicylates). The dietary approach should be to adopt a 'fresh foods' intake, and avoid convenience foods (as these foods are likely to contain additives/preservatives). Permitted foods include fresh meat and fish, eggs, milk and milk products with no artificial flavours, coffee, pastas and rice, white bread and plain cereals, permitted fruit and vegetables. Foods not permitted include fizzy drinks, beer, distilled drinks (whisky, vodka, gin), tea, wine, some fruits and vegetables, salad dressings and mayonnaise.
- The recording of foods in a diary together with a symptom record may raise awareness of possible 'trigger' foods. Management of asthma attacks will be important as they can increase histamine production (avoid red and white wine). Reduction of family stress (e.g. financial management) and the involvement in relaxation techniques are important lifestyle interventions. Use of alternative medications may be useful: anti-histamine preparations may cause drowsiness and are associated

Commentaries

with anergy, thus the patient may not eat, or be motivated to eat, particularly well. Vigilance with cosmetic products is important and liaison with pharmacy and checking labels on products will be valuable.

■ Practical advice includes the promotion of small, frequent meals, and care with preparation of food (avoiding skin contact) may be helpful. Dietary approaches should also concentrate on increasing intake of NSP (use of potatoes in jackets, and dried permitted fruit may be helpful) and promoting a regular meal pattern. A definitive, up-to-date list of 'foods permitted/foods to avoid' should be given to the patient to support advice. Monitoring of the client may return to the family doctor or care continued by the dietitian.

Case 32

Line of questioning in family members together with background research, reveals information that may assist in understanding about patterns of dietary intake, nutritional status and lifestyle factors longitudinally through a time frame:

■ relationship between dietary intake and lifestyle factors with expenditure on food, access to food, personal food preferences, world events (e.g. war) and significant trends in nutritional intake;
■ the changing role of diet from traditional feeding of families (earlier records) to more concerns about nutritional intake (government surveys, reports and development of policy);
■ disease patterning and life expectancy from the past to the present time;
■ the presence and influence of risk factors associated with the development of disease prevalence related to the time frame.

Case 33

Examination of the menus should consider the provision of meals:

■ in the context of the population group served (first class versus third class passengers);
■ in each of the population groups, does the menu provide sufficient variety to meet individual food preferences, cultural and religious preferences, physical needs (energy) and nutritional requirements?

Consideration may also be given to:

■ the contrast and comparison between the two menus (range of foods, quality of ingredients, and more especially the likely nutritional superiority of the third class menu);
■ the likely influence of the quality and quantity of nutrition of food provided by the menus in the context of health or health risk;
■ the menu items that are unfamiliar.

Case 34

- Significant points of the case include that Maria has a BMI of $17.3 \, kg/m^2$ and her current behaviour suggests she will continue to lose weight. She has had one medical emergency and is at high risk of heart failure. Re-feeding may be essential to reduce immediate risk but care must be taken to avoid development of re-feeding syndrome (unlikely in a specialist unit). The client is under pressure to maintain low body weight and may be unwilling to regain weight to remain professionally competitive. Further weight loss will most likely result in cognitive impairment and may compromise the effectiveness of psychotherapy. Blood work indicates malnutrition.

- The diagnosis of anorexia nervosa must be confirmed and assessment of the willingness to change behaviour ascertained. If the client is in the pre-contemplative stage, then raising awareness of risks may be motivating. Assessment of weight and BMI may be considered weekly. Blood work may be routinely monitored and guidelines for re-feeding followed. Diet histories before development of, and during the acute phase of anorexia nervosa may be useful. Assessing knowledge of the link between low body weight and malnutrition may be helpful. Assessment of symptoms is routine (see Cases 16 and 17); assessment of cognitive function (memory, concentration) is important. A bone density scan may be considered. A CBT approach is appropriate. Biochemical parameters may be managed by appropriate supplementation. A full psychological assessment may give further insight as to cause and likely treatment plan for the client.

- Short-term goals include prevention of further weight loss and the establishment of regular and sensible eating. This may involve waiting until the client is ready to change behaviour. Increasing Maria's knowledge of nutrition in association with key points of her condition may be important. Treatment may focus on what concerns the client most (motivation). Cognitive function will be improved by re-feeding as will resolution of some of the symptoms. Weight regain of the order of 0.5–1.0 kg/week may be the target by optimising food intake and reducing obsessional physical activity.

- In the longer term, goals include: maintenance of weight gain and reinforcement of regular eating pattern. The variety and range of foods consumed should be increased with the ultimate aim of achieving a BMI within the healthy range. In addition, achieving consistent and normal clinical chemistry (haemoglobin and cholesterol) is a goal. A relapse prevention strategy must be in place and a sensible approach to all aspects of diet and lifestyle encouraged.

- Education is the key to providing reassurance and nutritional guidelines communicated through a healthy eating model of dietary intervention. A discussion about weight, starvation and the likely consequences to health may be appropriate. An explanation of rapid weight gain initially may assist in the client engaging with treatment. Management necessitates a client-centred approach with negotiated and agreed targets (meal plan, weekly targets, energy intake increments across time) together with keeping of records (food and mood diaries).

■ Monitoring may include knowledge and understanding assessment, exploring attitude to weight and shape, assessment of food intake (diaries), assessment of motivation at each session and monitoring of weight and BMI (weekly). Monitoring of clinical chemistry (significant parameters), blood pressure and cardiovascular parameters may be helpful. Towards the end of a six-month period, or when a satisfactory outcome is reached, plans should be put into place for a relapse prevention strategy.

■ Significant challenges presented in this case centre on the client's possible resistance to change behaviour and the likely cognitive impairment which may be compromised by weight loss thus hampering prognosis from psychotherapy. If the client continues to lose weight, she will be further medically compromised and enteral feeding will become a necessity. If consent from the client is not given, then the MDT may decide whether to feed or not (under the terms of the Mental Health Act).

Case 35

■ During the run-up period to surgery, the intake of a normal diet (hospital diet) would be encouraged and the main goal will be to ensure that the client meets nutritional requirements. His weight needs to be ascertained so that energy and protein requirements can be calculated to achieve optimum nutritional status. Food and drink intake needs to be monitored to assess whether requirements are being met. The patient may need to be counselled on carbohydrate loading prior to surgery as part of the ERAS protocol, to prevent insulin resistance following surgery.

■ Nutritional goals after the surgery are similar to the pre-operative ones, except that intake may shift towards a sip-feeding regimen (3 sip feeds/d) from day 1, providing the patient does not develop an ileus. Post-operatively, there may be a huge emphasis on nutritional support, especially if a period of radiotherapy is anticipated.

■ If the patient has a stoma placed, then this would result in a modified diet. Meeting nutritional goals, however, is still paramount with dietary intake (food record charts) and blood biochemistry monitoring. Gradually, sip feeds may be reduced and replaced with snacks (between meals) and fortified food (together with a vitamin and mineral supplement) with the option to continue sip feeds as necessary. The patient may be weighed twice weekly.

Case 36

■ Initial impressions of the case strongly suggest that the client has compromised nutritional status, due to poor dietary intake resulting from difficulty in food provision and preparation, reduced appetite and altered taste/food preference, difficulty with mastication and swallowing, social isolation, financial circumstances, age and impaired cognitive status.

∎ Assessment parameters include BMI (15.9 kg/m^2), weight loss (15%), and a probable high risk nutritional screening score. His requirements can be calculated using predictive equations: energy: BMR (8.3 × 45) + 820 = 1194 kcal; addition of 400 kcal to promote weight gain = 1594 kcal and adjustment for PAL = 1594 × 1.4 = 2231 kcal/d. He has protein depletion, and an intake of 70 g/d should meet his requirement (0.25 gN × 45 × 6.25 = 70 g protein).

∎ Short-term goals should focus on meeting requirements, and basing the intake on fortified hospital diet together with additional snacks between meals. An appropriate oral nutritional supplement should be prescribed, depending on oral intake. The patient needs to be monitored (food record intake chart) and encouraged (and prompted) to eat (especially snacks).

∎ If full meals are eaten, the hospital diet may provide about 1500–1800 kcal/d. This may be fortified to add additional energy, by appropriate use of butter, margarine, cheese, milk powder and other commercial agents (e.g. Pro-Cal, Maxijul). The range of food items may necessarily limit the use of these. Energy intake can be boosted by appropriate use of snacks. Prescribing an oral supplement (2 × 200 ml of sip feed/d) would assist in meeting increased nutritional requirements; these should be administered to take account of taste, volume and cost of the supplement and it may be worth experimenting with a variety of supplements to find the most appropriate for the patient.

∎ In the longer term, goals include the smooth transition from hospital to home and perhaps arranging support via social services, including provision of meals-on-wheels. Prescription of nutritional supplements should continue at home until such time as the nutritional status improves clinical outcome.

∎ Monitoring at ward level will mean liaising with ward staff (observation and record keeping) to explore food and drink intake over time. Monitoring food intake in a demented patient presents a challenge: for those clients who are relatively independent eaters, you may have to rely on the patient's memory or work out the difference between what is presented and what is left or rejected. For the dependent eater, records are easier and will be kept by the carer or individual responsible for feeding the client.

Case 37

∎ Short-term goals centre on providing nutritional requirements via nasogastric feeding. Longer-term goals include maintaining an appropriate weight and muscle mass, which can be monitored using weight parameters and arm anthropometry.

Commentaries

- Nutritional requirements may be estimated or calculated using predictive equations to include baseline data (weight 54 kg and height 1.60 m). Energy requirements may be met by: BMR = (14.8 × 54) + 485 kcal, the addition of a mobility factor (10%), the addition of a stress factor (fever) of 25% and a factor to account for ventilation (40%) = 1284 + 963 = 2250 kcal/d. Protein requirements may be met be supplying 67–85 g/d (hypermetabolic patients require an additional 5–25%). Fluid requirements may be met by 35 ml × 54 = 1900 ml + 110 ml (pyrexia) = 2100 ml/d.
- Monitoring of the feed should include urine and blood electrolytes, and the aim should be to increase the energy density of the feed to 1.5 kcal/ml, depending on blood test results. There is no reason to suspect re-feeding syndrome.
- Monitoring should include arm anthropometry (MAMC, TSF, to assess LBM) and weight (fat stores can be assessed if unable to accurately weigh the patient). Clinical chemistry should be monitored, at least until the patient is clinically stable.

Case 38

- Initial impressions of the case suggest a well-orientated and busy woman. She is a weight loser and likely to have >10% weight loss (in two months) and may be malnourished. She has side-effects of chemotherapy.
- Eyeball assessment indicates underweight and malnutrition. Further assessments are required, and include: BMI, MUAC and TSF measurements and comparison with normal reference ranges. Baseline data can be used to monitor nutritional status over time. It may be useful to check other medications and monitor risk of re-feeding syndrome.
- Short-term issues include: reducing the effects of chemotherapy (tailored dietary advice), targeting advice about managing nausea (use of anti-emetics, use of cold food, benefit of fresh air, trying alternative protein-containing foods, mouth care and oral hygiene, use of sharp-tasting drinks and sweet foods) and concentrating on foods that she enjoys. Poor appetite may be managed by use of steroids. Clinical priorities clearly centre on avoidance of further weight loss and meeting dietary requirements (protein, energy, electrolytes, minerals and micronutrients and fluid). The client may be advised about food hygiene. Aggressive use of food fortification and food supplements may be considered useful to meet requirements but against monitoring for re-feeding syndrome. Exploration of social circumstances may be useful (Is she too tired to cook? Can she eat at the bowls club?).
- In the longer term, clinical goals include achieving a healthy weight and preventing malnutrition. Prophylactic healthy eating advice against further cancers may be useful. The client needs to engage with care and therefore needs to be taught to recognise and respond to changes in well-being and nutritional status. The client needs to re-engage with social activities.

Commentaries

- Implementation of dietary intervention rests on classification of weight lost (>10% in three months) or BMI (>18.5 kg/m²) and warrants nutritional support to prevent malnutrition. Use of food fortification, oral nutritional supplements or even ANS is indicated. Actual requirements should be calculated; there is a need to obtain further information (age, weight, weight history and activity factor). Approaches to ensure the client meets requirements are crucial: making suitable food selection, fortifying foods where possible and choice of appropriate nutritional supplements (flavour, temperature, ward and patient education to optimise intake, liaison with the Catering department). Nocturnal feeding may be appropriate (to provide 1000 kcal), but there is a need to assess oral intake (energy, protein, micronutrients, fluid and NSP) and aim to meet nutritional requirements. A low volume, high energy/protein/NSP feed may be useful; give extra fluid (water) to meet fluid requirements or use of a standard feed (1000 kcal/1 kcal/ml) may be appropriate depending on the patient's voluntary intake, tolerance and blood biochemistry.
- Monitoring and evaluation should begin daily, reducing to twice weekly and then three to six monthly, and may include: weight, MAC and TSF, gastrointestinal function, symptom record and any changes to the clinical condition and significant clinical chemistry. Social circumstances and compliance issues require monitoring.

Case 39

- Assessment of dietary intake is essential to establish some baseline information. A 24-hr recall of intake may be sufficient; a 72 hr intake may provide a better history from which to establish information. Other assessments may include: arm anthropometry (MAC and TSF) and grip strength, usual diabetic parameters (e.g. HbA_{1c}) and parameters indicative of alcohol consumption (triglyceride and GTT levels). Assessment of enzyme use and practice may be helpful.
- Regardless of how long ago the patient trained as a dietitian, she should still be aware of the longer-term implications and complications of poor diabetic control. There is a need to find out what she is interested in socially, and perhaps try to relate this to long-term complications (e.g. reading and retinopathy). To prompt use of pancreatic enzyme supplements, the client should be encouraged to take these *with* food (and snacks) and store them beside her cutlery.
- The major nutritional aim is to improve nutritional status by reinforcing healthy eating, conforming with clinical guidelines for diabetic people (Diabetes UK). This may result in an improvement in dietary intake (guided by baseline dietary assessment), an increase in use of pancreatic enzymes (Creon) and insulin accordingly. The client should be reviewed locally at clinic and the necessary support given. For example, if misuse of alcohol is suspected, then the patient should be referred to local support networks.

Commentaries

■ The case may present with some difficulty: one should not assume that a dietitian who trained some time ago would be familiar with the specific aspects of contemporary (and evidence-based) dietary intervention, especially when the case suggests some compliance issues (adherence to dose and intake of enzymes, possible alcohol misuse and reclusive behaviour).

Case 40

■ The case presents a very underweight, older woman with a serious diagnosis and difficult social situation. The patient, in light of imminent surgery and severe underweight, may benefit from 7–10 days of pre-operative nutritional support (NICE 2006) and her case needs to be discussed with the surgeon and nursing staff. Nutritional support may be accomplished by provision of high energy/high protein meals, drinks and snacks together with appropriate additional supplementation. Nasogastric feeding may be considered if her oral intake is very poor, though she is at risk of re-feeding syndrome. It is unclear whether the patient has been underweight for some time or if weight loss is recent; the latter is of greater concern, and needs to be ascertained. Baseline clinical chemistry should be assessed and caution should be exercised if considering supplementation or nasogastric feeding. Biochemistry, fluid balance and clinical status should be carefully monitored (NICE, 2006 and PENG, 2004).

■ As is standard practice, energy requirements should be calculated using predictive equations: BMR = $(9.8 \times 43.5) + 624 = 1050$ kcal/d, which is adjusted for stress and activity/DIT. Weight gain adjustment of energy intake may not be wise (risk of re-feeding syndrome). NICE guidelines suggest restricting total energy intake to 10 kcal/kg in patients at high risk of re-feeding syndrome, but this would represent an intake of 435 kcal/d, which may be a questionable intake (a good practice guide, but not based on random controlled trials). The patient shows interest in hospital diet, suggesting that weight loss is due to poor intake (probably because of lack of interest in preparing food). It may be useful to consider first, offering a palatable, nutritious hospital diet together with appropriate use of supplements. A dietary history may provide information on which to base a reasonable dietary prescription to provide a modest increase to her current dietary intake. Thereafter, intake may be escalated (with monitoring) to a point which promotes pre-operative weight gain. It would be important to discuss the risk of early versus delayed surgery with the medical team as an improvement in her nutritional status will take some time to achieve. NICE guidelines also recommend that B vitamins and electrolytes supplementation should be considered in patients with a BMI <16 kg/m². Re-feeding syndrome is associated with fluid overload and fluid balance should be carefully monitored.

■ Height, weight and BMI should always be recorded together with an account of oral intake.

- This patient requires careful monitoring including anthropometry, dietary intake, full biochemical profile, clinical condition and haematology according to best practice guidelines (NICE, 2006 and PENG, 2004).

Case 41

- The initial view of the case is of a client with long-standing bowel history and who has disease-related malnutrition and associated weight loss. Aggressive feeding may increase the risk of developing the re-feeding syndrome.
- Baseline assessment measures should include assessment of actual weight, BMI and percentage weight loss. Baseline biochemistry parameters are important and may include determination of LFTs, urine and blood electrolytes, plasma/serum phosphorus and magnesium, fluid status and renal function. Gastrointestinal function may be reviewed as the patient is likely to have a nil-by-mouth period, and because of the surgical procedure. Protein, energy and fluid requirements need to be estimated.
- The short-term goal for priority is to provide nutritional support to meet nutritional requirements, either via oral nutrition (gluten-free, fortified diet together with sip feeds), by using enteral feeding (if unlikely to meet nutritional requirements by oral nutrition) or by parenteral nutrition (if unlikely to meet nutritional requirements by above means, or if the gut is not working or is not accessible).
- In the longer term, nutritional status needs to be maintained (protein and energy) and gluten-free dietary advice given to reinforce diet priorities (adequate mineral and vitamin content). Prescription of both gluten-free products and oral nutritional supplements should continue as required, until the patient is able to tolerate full oral diet.
- Monitoring should occur weekly (in hospital) to ensure appropriate nutritional support is delivered to meet clinical aims. This may involve regular evaluation of blood plasma/serum biochemistry (albumin, urea, creatinine, potassium, magnesium, phosphorus, LFTs) together with fluid balance and weight change data. The dietitian should be vigilant for signs of the re-feeding syndrome. Monitoring can revert to four-weekly evaluations after discharge and continue until optimal nutritional status is reached. The patient may be reviewed as often as necessary so that the dietitian is confident that the patient has a good grasp of a basic gluten-free diet. The GP needs to receive care documentation outlining the treatment plan and outcomes.

Case 42

- The patient should be advised to follow a healthy, energy-deficit diet to encourage weight loss and assist with reducing pain (weight bearing on arthritic joints). The diet may be constructed on a modified BoGH and the energy prescription based on BMR and PAL. The energy prescription

Commentaries

may be calculated: BMR = $(8.7 \times 80) + 696 = 1525$ kcal, together with PAL: 1525×1.56 (light activity) = 2379 kcal/d. To encourage weight loss, and with the introduction of a deficit of 5–700 kcal, the diet may be based on about 1800 kcal/d.

■ The healthy eating advice should be reinforced with the need to include omega-3 fatty acids in the diet (e.g. use of oily fish) or use of an appropriate supplement (to improve stiffness and joint pain). Inclusion of starchy carbohydrates at each meal is important (to reduce post-prandial slump and for slow release of energy). Healthy eating snack ideas will provide practical help with managing hunger between meals (e.g. fruit). The encouragement of exercise is important, but will be limited to what the client can manage comfortably, but may include chair exercises, daily walks and swimming. Suspected lactose intolerance may be investigated and the use of appropriate intervention established if a formal diagnosis is made. The patient may continue, if desired, to avoid specific foods. It may be that the patient has self-diagnosed this, given her interest in alternative therapy.

Case 43

■ Initial assessment may begin with a baseline dietary assessment (e.g. a 24-hr recall) to reveal the general impression of the intake. A more detailed dietary assessment may be warranted, perhaps with use of a seven-day diary. It will be useful to link this with a symptom record.

■ The main challenge presented in this case is the difficulty in proving that particular foods are causing symptoms when it may be a coincidental association.

■ Assessment should include clinical chemistry (serum vitamin B_{12}) due to the site of the condition, and calcium levels (one of the aims will be to reduce the risk of osteoporosis). The client should be encouraged to consume about 1500 mg calcium per day, and the dietary intake may need to be supported by the use of supplements.

■ Short-term goals should include meeting requirements for protein and energy and fat soluble vitamin intake is of key interest (because of the self-imposed restriction of dietary fat). Given the BMI, the quality of the diet may be more important than meeting macronutrient intakes. A high intake of dietary fat is sometimes associated with increasing the risk of inflammation in patients with Crohn's disease, and it may be useful to explore what the patient perceives as a 'fat-free diet'. Often strictures occur in the terminal ileum and lead to pain when eating some foods high in NSP – this may be perceived as intolerance to wheat and may need investigation. Rather more controversially perhaps, a complete elemental diet (tailored to meet nutritional requirements) that is hypoallergenic, could be considered. This may allow the patient to re-introduce foods sequentially to give an indication of specific tolerance.

Commentaries

Case 44

- This case presents as a patient with long-standing type 1 diabetes whose principal health concern is his weight (he is currently obese, if assumed of average height) and the associated health risks associated with over-weight. Clearly, intervention must centre on weight management and general advice, such as ensuring that intake of salt and alcohol are within recommended target levels. Physical activity levels will depend on whether he participates in training or engages in other forms of exercise.
- Initial assessment should look at all routine parameters studied in the care of a diabetic patient and consider these with regard to target levels. Intervention should be planned, or reinforced, using these parameters as a reference point. A particular focus of dietary investigation may be useful (dietary history) to obtain information on how and why the client's weight has crept up over time.
- Short-term goals include maintaining appropriate glycaemic control and establishing a plan for reduction in weight, based on an energy-deficit, healthy eating intake. Dietary reinforcement may be required (depend-ing on actual intake) to firmly establish the intake on healthy eating principles. The client's energy intake to assist weight reduction may be calculated, or simply adjusted from his current baseline diet (e.g. encour-age smaller portions, reduction in intake of alcohol). An appropriate intake of energy may be about 2500–2700 kcal/d, based on BMR (11.6 × 103.9 + 879 = 2084 kcal), PAL (1.55 × 2084 = 3231 kcal) and to include an energy deficit factor of 5–700 kcal/d. Appropriate dietary advice may include reinforcement of the quantity and type of dietary fat to be eaten.
- In the longer term, goals should focus on sustaining good glycaemic control whilst maintaining a programme of steady, slow and sustained weight loss. The client may be followed up at a general/diabetic clinic or by the practice nurse. Monitoring should consist of comparing routine diabetic parameters with clinic and weight reduction targets. Waist cir-cumference may be the preferred method of monitoring progress in weight management. With regular follow up at the diabetic clinic dietary changes and insulin regimens can be kept under review.

Case 45

- Initial impressions suggest that this case is a typical presentation of prob-able non-organic failure to thrive, poor meal patterns exacerbated by ADHD and possible poor pattern of growth. The meals pattern may represent what works best for the family situation, consisting of quick meals. Meals are difficult times; food is often rejected.
- Assessment may begin with investigating the meal pattern and quantities of food consumed. It may be important to establish a detailed record of intake, but even a quick dietary summary may give useful information (quantities and types of food chosen may be evident).

- Short-term goals include improving quality of food and drink consumed at meals and snacks. In particular, improving vitamin and mineral centent of the intake is a priority, in addition to ensuring adequate energy. Establishing a meal and snack routine as a habitual pattern is important. It may be useful to consider a short-term diet supplement to assist with weight gain if weight has fallen across centile lines.
- In the longer term, nutritional goals may aim for healthy eating, using a family approach. The intake of processed and junk foods should be reduced.
- Approaches and implementation of goals may include: aiming to meet dietary reference values for the age range for energy and protein, encouraging the child to consume five portions of fruit and vegetables a day and encouraging an intake of oily fish to improve omega-3 fatty acid status. It is important to review all aspects of diet against the current evidence base for diet in ADHD.
- Monitoring and evaluation may include review of diet and diet quality as changes are implemented. It may be important to review anthropometry from baseline and review assessments as the dietary changes are implemented (perhaps every eight weeks). Compliance may be an issue and it will be important to engage the client with the changes made to diet so that he may understand why the changes are being made and that he can be involved with negotiating changes. The school and others involved in his life need to be consistent with approaches taken. Activity patterns may also be useful and encourage the child to get involved (activity diary).
- The case presents some key issues: it may be helpful to establish whether there is a non-organic cause and explore the school's ability to provide adequate supervision. Individual monitoring may require that the school has a 'Statement of Special Educational Needs' so that a named individual has specific responsibility for this case. It may be useful to explore the client's weight/growth history more closely (perhaps even anecdotally) together with maternal height and the family's socio-economic status.

Case 46

- Mrs Montgomery presents as a reasonably fit, 85 year old who is beginning to struggle cognitively. She lives in a care home and has a good appetite, but is beginning to lose weight and is at risk of malnutrition. She needs assistance to prevent further decline (especially with a progressive, neurological condition). The client's short-term goal centres on maintaining weight status and avoiding weight loss. The nutritional care plan needs to be reassessed frequently, to take account of poor cognitive function and appetite, and should include improvement of the nutritional quality of meals/snacks (fortification). The use of supplements should be reviewed, perhaps to reduce the number and replace with a higher energy, fat emulsion-based type if dietary intake is good. Intake and weight parameters should be monitored.

■ Mrs Hamilton presents as a frail 84 year old who has poor mobility, is in hospital and has a poor appetite. Several acute factors are contributing to malnutrition; the patient is likely to have already lost weight. She needs intensive dietetic input. A short-term goal is to minimise the risk of further weight loss. Aggressive feeding may be considered and may involve the use of daily nutritional supplements (depending on the severity of the resection) or nasogastric feeding. A high-protein, energy-dense diet may need to rely on use of liquids or a liquidised diet. Monitoring will focus on weight parameters, tolerance of supplements/oral diet and intake. Assessment will include review of appetite, factors following resection of the tongue, such as chewing ability and risk assessment of weight loss following treatment (e.g. radiotherapy).

■ Clearly the main contrast focuses on the baseline fitness of the two patients and the ethical consideration of the extent to which aggressive feeding should be implemented.

Case 47

■ This elderly woman's physical symptoms (hacking cough and infection) will be making her feel unwell and exhausted. It is understandable that she takes little interest in food, as she is unlikely to enjoy either shopping for, or preparing, meals. Infection will induce an acute phase protein response and increase her nutritional requirements but also means that she is unlikely to gain substantially (increasing muscle mass) even from establishing nutritional support. It is important that these infections are effectively managed to help improve nutritional status. Her husband's desire to lose weight, and the tension this may bring, will make it hard for her to have energy-dense snacks at home and the couple will need careful counselling and appropriate social support to help manage this situation.

■ The short-term goal will be to introduce nutritional support cautiously as this patient is at high risk of re-feeding syndrome (with a BMI <16 kg/m^2). The dietitian may try to ensure that the patient has help with shopping and cooking; advice on provision of appropriate meals is important. The patient may be advised to have small, frequent meals to start with, and nutritional supplements may be given as tolerated. Close monitoring is important to ensure reasonable compliance with the intake. Nasogastric feeding may be considered depending on progress with oral intake and will require community nursing support (assuming the patient is at home).

■ In the longer term, goals include the priority of achieving and maintaining nutritional status through: appropriate liaison with the medical team regarding management of the clinical condition and pain relief and liaison with nursing staff regarding social care arrangements and provision of additional help (e.g. meals-on-wheels). Nutritional requirements should be re-calculated periodically, and should promote weight gain (if clinical status improves). Sip feeds should be given between meals;

perhaps consideration of fruit-based feeds may be more appropriate, to counter the problem of phlegm production (milk-based foods). Tolerance and preference of feeds must always determine products selected. The evidence for intake of feeds with a higher fat:carbohydrate ratio remains unconvincing. The client may benefit from a discussion/advice about use and sources of high-energy foods (e.g. whole milk/products) as well as shopping advice and how to compromise with husband's needs and food preferences. Monitoring should be frequent, and perhaps daily to begin with (food and fluid intake, clinical chemistry and micronutrient status).

Case 48

■ The case presents some challenges. It is unclear if the patient is malnourished (the use of BMI alone may be limited in reaching a decision). The absence of a weight history or knowledge of usual weight also hampers forming a decision about nutritional status, and may be something to explore with the client. If there has been recent weight loss, it may suggest the presence of diabetes or an alcohol-related liver disease. The client presents with an erratic pattern of eating and preferred foods are high in salt and saturated fat, but there is a need to explore quantities and how consistent the intake is over a week. There is an opportunity to enhance nutritional status by improving the quality of the intake and make suggestions about lifestyle change to support the client. There may be motivation issues and the client has to be ready to change dietary and lifestyle behaviour. It may be useful to enlist the help of support services (smoking cessation service, alcohol rehabilitation, engagement in light physical exercise).

■ Assessment may include a general look at the client's medical history together with a full inspection of clinical chemistry (LFTs, blood pressure, serum lipid profile and blood glucose). There is a need to exclude diagnoses of liver involvement and diabetes. A screen for cardiovascular risk factors may be useful. The BMI indicates underweight but it will be useful to consider any recent and significant weight loss. Muscle anthropometry assessment will be useful to compare with reference standards. The classification of the client being 'too thin' should be explored in light of data collected. Waist circumference measurement may be considered (ongoing monitoring). Assumptions about dietary intake need to be confirmed by diet assessment and probing for quality of diet and meal patterns will be useful. Estimates of total energy/protein intake will form the basis of intervention diet and advice and may be elicited using diet history or food diary. Estimates of sodium intake will also inform if this is a diet priority.

■ Short-term goals will be informed by assessment of the case. If assessment suggests poor nutritional intake/status, then the priority will be to improve lean body mass/relative fat mass using usual diet as a basis for intervention (high energy/high protein intake). It will be useful to consider if requirements can be achieved with normal diet, and will be preferable to use nutritional supplements. There should be a switch away from saturated fats to an intake rich in MUFA sources of fat, together with a reduction in salt intake. The use of a high sugar intake may be considered. Another priority will be to improve variety of the diet intake and make full use of all the food groups. The practicalities of carrying a breakfast and lunch to work may be discussed together with encouraging general dietary improvements, such as including fruit scones, teacakes spread with appropriate fat (MUFA based) and jam and incorporation of more fruit, fruit milkshakes and smoothie-type drinks (with appropriate ice-cream), lean meat/oily fish and salad sandwiches (on wholegrain bread). Eating jacket potatoes with appropriate fillings (e.g. tuna and low fat mayonnaise) may be discussed. Attention should focus on easily made and eaten items, and ones that may not attract derision from his work-mates. The client may benefit from guidance on preparation of simple evening meals, such as poached eggs and baked beans (low salt) on toast (MUFA spread), or consider buying healthy option foods/ready meals with added vegetables/salad (olive oil dressings). Key messages will be emphasis on sugar, MUFA fats and reducing salt intake. Dietary advice may be based on a healthy eating model (e.g. BoGH). There is also a need for the client to engage in light physical exercise, and this should be negotiated at a first appointment. Advice on how to interpret food labels will be useful. The family doctor should be informed of the intervention strategy.

■ In the longer term, goals include regular contact with health promotion dietitians in primary care who will reinforce dietary priorities (especially alcohol and salt intake, and the quality of fat in the diet). Risk factors associated with these may form the basis of discussion at review appointments and will provide motivation. Lifestyle factors also need emphasis (regular eating, regular exercise and diet moderation). Support services may be useful. The family doctor should be kept informed of progress.

■ Close monitoring may be useful and the client may be reviewed within two weeks. Comparison of nutritional status with baseline data is paramount to demonstrate change/improvement, which may very well be motivational. Compliance and access to support services may be important to monitor.

■ A significant challenge of the case will be to provide enough energy/protein to meet requirements without promoting intake of dietary fat. In addition, lifestyle change and a switch to planning his dietary intakes much more, may be difficult to achieve unless motivated. His social life involves the use of alcohol, which may be difficult to change.

Case 49

■ Initial data indicates 30% burn injury, which is a shock burn. He is a fit, young man, and may have significant LBM, which will lead to rapid weight loss in the initial phase of treatment (he will be fairly immobile). He is likely to have high requirements and it will be difficult to meet these by oral diet. He is first seen on day 4, when catabolism is already in progress.

■ Baseline assessment includes a BMI of 29.4 kg/m^2, but he may be muscular. A 30% total burns surface area means that he may have functional difficulties (unable to sit, feed himself and walk due to large bulky dressings at joints). His current oral intake is 800 kcal which is insufficient to meet requirements.

■ Short-term priorities include increasing his nutritional intake to meet requirements; this is best achieved using a nasogastric feed (he struggles to consume 800 kcal/d). The major goal is to minimise weight loss (he will receive physiotherapy to maintain function). The timing of feeds should allow for repeated trips to theatre (wound debridements, skin grafting and change of dressings) and periods of nil-by-mouth. The use of energy-dense/high protein oral supplements is indicated in conjunction with tube feed and oral diet.

■ In the longer term, it is important to recognise that the client is likely to have a prolonged recovery period; burns patients may still be having surgery several years after the initial injury. The client will need to follow an energy-dense/high protein diet until his burns have healed and he has regained sufficient weight to give a satisfactory BMI. He will not regain his former muscle tone until he has resumed an active lifestyle.

■ Calculated requirements: energy = (15.1 × 85) + 692 kcal = 1976 kcal + 20% stress (burns) + 15% (activity) = 2667 kcal/d. 20% of energy to be supplied by protein = 133 g protein. Fluid requirements = 35 ml × 85 = 2975 ml fluid. Using a combination of oral and enteral feeds, assuming oral diet provides 15–20 g protein, 1000 ml Jevity Plus (56 g protein/1200 kcal), 600 ml Fortimel (60 g protein/600 kcal) and oral diet (? protein/800 kcal) provide requirements. If oral intake falls, then the feed can be increased. Calogen may be used to provide additional energy if the patient has no oral intake at all. Some feeds provide a higher N:energy ratio and may be considered.

■ The patient will probably need to be reviewed three times every week initially, and possibly daily depending on toleration of the feeding regimen, theatre trips, etc. There is a need to monitor food record charts, fluid balance charts, weight status and blood biochemistry. Anthropometry will be difficult to complete initially because of the burned areas but this may be useful in recovery phase and outpatient settings.

■ Particular management issues centre around the time available to feed the patient – big burns take several hours to be dressed and can be very painful. The other concern may be that the patient was health conscious prior to the injury and it may be difficult to encourage an energy-dense intake orally.

Case 50

■ This is a case of a woman who is a long-standing diabetic and is currently not on oral hypoglycaemic agents, perhaps because of her lack of attendance at a diabetic clinic. She has clearly been struggling for some time and has some degree of malnutrition (low iron and albumin status, weight loss). Weight loss may be as a result of poor diabetes control and home situation. Dietary intake may have been hampered by problems at home (not being able to prepare food, reduced taste sensation, depression and possibly limited support from her family).

■ On admission, nutritional risk should be assessed using a dedicated tool (e.g. MUST) and dietetic intervention will be determined by the score achieved. Given the weight loss (8 kg), together with the fact that her weight was once normal, this may classify her as medium or high risk (of malnutrition). Treatment will be based on food record charts; offering extra snacks to support dietary intake is preferable to offering nutritional supplements (refer to local protocol). Initially, screening should be repeated weekly.

■ If the screening tool score is high (indicating high risk) then the dietitian will be informed, requirements calculated and an appropriate regimen implemented. Energy and protein requirements will be calculated using suitable predictive formulae: energy: weight (kg) $\times$ 9.8 + 624 kcal, with the addition of a stress factor (10%) as she is bed bound, together with an additional 500 kcal/d to promote weight increase. Protein: weight (kg) $\times$ 0.17 = x gN $\times$ 6.25 = x g protein/d.

■ Renal status should be checked as well as degree of glycaemic control. Staff may be reluctant to continue nutritional supplements if required, as they may be perceived to raise blood glucose levels. It is clearly important, therefore, to stress the need to tighten glycaemic control. The diabetes team should be involved in this patient's management, and will probably need insulin initially to improve glycaemic control quickly. Insulin therapy may also be required post-discharge, and should feature as part of discharge arrangements and documentation. It may be wise to get input from the rheumatology team.

■ Short-term goals will centre on improving oral intake to: improve wound healing, optimise recovery, optimise glycaemic control, optimise nutritional status and reduce the risk of hypos. Longer-term nutritional goals include extending the short-term goals to include: promotion of a varied diet based on the BoGH, meeting nutritional requirements, experience enjoyment through eating and incorporating the occasional treat. Medically, goals will include maintaining glycaemic control with regular monitoring (HbA$_{1c}$).

Case 51

■ Clinical chemistry is consistent with the presence of ascites (low albumin and sodium concentrations). Liver involvement is suggested by other clinical data: prothrombin time is prolonged, and may be as a result of poor liver synthesis of clotting factors; bilirubin concentration is high and presumably accounts for the jaundice; LFTs are abnormal and GGT is high due to fatty infiltration secondary to alcohol misuse. Haemoglobin and potassium concentrations are low, and suggest that the patient is anaemic; there is a need to consider checking serum folate and vitamin B_{12} status, together with MCV.

■ Short-term nutritional goals include implementation of a low sodium diet (80–100 mmol/d) together with a fluid restriction. His dietary intake should be nutrient dense (food and snacks) and consideration needs to be given to the use of sip feeds to support his oral intake. Monitoring should include dietary intake (food record charts), daily weight and MAMC and girth measurements every two months. In the longer term, the aim will be to encourage healthy eating and to establish regular meal planning in the context of a NAS diet.

■ Assessment of nutritional requirements needs to take account of 4 litres fluid as ascites (he has de-compensated liver disease). Weight = 73 kg (includes wet weight) − 4 kg, to result in a dry weight of 69 kg. Energy requirements can be calculated using 25–45 kcal/kg/d or BMR (+30–40%). With a dry weight of 69 kg, his energy requirements are 1725–3105 kcal/d or 1666 + 500 kcal (30% stress) = 2166 kcal/d. Experience perhaps suggests that an intake of 2200 kcal/d is appropriate. Protein requirements: N = 0.25 × 69 = 17 gN (×6.25) = 108 g protein/d. The key element in this case is monitoring once a regimen is established; MAMC and grip strength are important. Ordinary hospital diet together with food fortification may be the most appropriate solution, as extra fluid coming from sip feeds may not be advisable (also, no soups from the hospital menu).

■ Practical advice should prioritise the consumption of a high protein, energy-dense NAS diet, and follow-up is crucial to prevent relapse. Liaison with the local alcohol team is important if available; success may depend on how receptive the client is to this form of rehabilitation and changing of habits.

■ Follow-up at a gastroenterological clinic may include monitoring of neurological signs, numbness in hands/feet, weight, the presence of heartburn, memory and vision. Clearly, a management priority is cessation of drinking alcohol, and an appropriate counselling strategy should be established by the alcohol support nurse.

Case 52

■ This is a case of a woman with a history of persistent gastrointestinal problems. She may be at risk of malnutrition since her symptoms appear to be deteriorating and it is not entirely clear whether she has lost weight prior to admission. Symptoms appear to resolve after rehydration. Key points to address include weight loss and vomiting.

■ Short-term nutritional goals centre on ensuring that the patient meets nutritional requirements prior to partial gastrectomy. Prevention of further weight loss is important. This may be achieved with establishment of a high protein/high energy diet, using appropriate advice together with information on nutritional supplements and how to meet fluid requirements (to stem dehydration as a result of vomiting). It may be useful to advise the client to eat little and often and to regularly assess tolerance of foods, textures and fluids. Regular use of anti-emetics and/ or prokinetics will assist with gastric motility and reduce vomiting (e.g. metoclopramide, domperidone).

■ Longer-term priorities include monitoring for signs of post-operative dumping syndrome and pernicious anaemia and taking action with appropriate advice and medical intervention (injections of vitamin B_{12}). Continuing with nutritional supplements is important (assuming tolerance) if the patient can tolerate normal diet and fluids. Monitoring blood work is also important.

■ Monitoring weight pre- and post-surgery is important and there should be follow-up in clinic at four weeks post surgery. Bowel habits should be monitored together with full blood counts to assess iron status.

■ The case presents some difficulty in that height and weight are not given; the amount of weight loss will determine how aggressive nutritional support should be.

Case 53

■ Initial impressions indicate that the client is gaining weight too quickly and that energy intake is likely to be exceeding requirements. The client is consuming only two meals a day and needs advice regarding constipation and anaemia.

■ Assessment of the client may include: investigation of causes of weight gain and the need to check further weight gain, exploration of the carbohydrate load and the extent of intake of traditional dietary items, examination of diet patterns when her partner is not at home (does she eat well?) and assessment of what the client perceives as *too much weight*.

■ Short-term dietary goals include: regulation of portion sizes and establishment of a regular meal pattern, reduction of intake of foods and drinks high in sugar, reduction in total dietary energy intake to closer match requirements, to give dietary advice about constipation and anaemia, minimising weight gain without compromising nutritional status and achieving normal blood glucose levels to reduce the risk of having a large-for-date baby.

■ Longer-term goals may include increasing and sustaining physical exercise, reinforcing nutritional advice for pregnancy and gestational diabetes and maintaining the motivation to support weight management.

■ Dietary intervention would centre on an energy-deficit dietary intake, perhaps based on a predictive equation: BMR = (14.8 × 80.2) + 487 = 1673 kcal, PAL = 1673 × 1.4 = 2342 kcal/d (assuming non-active and light occupational activity). Current energy intake exceeds requirements and if continued will result in persistent tendency to gain weight through remainder of the pregnancy. It may be prudent to implement modest control of energy intake to about 2000 kcal/d.

■ Monitoring and evaluation may consist of: regular weight checks at every clinic visit (when seen by the diabetes team), repeat blood work (to check anaemia status), monthly HbA_{1c} assessment, regular assessment of bowel habit (self-reporting by patient) and commencement of home blood glucose testing (and keeping a diary record). The client needs to be aware, at some point, of the increased risk of developing type 2 diabetes in future and be informed of ways to assist risk reduction.

Case 54

■ The case presents as an older woman who has a busy life and has recently lost weight. She has become hypertensive, seeks help from her GP and is diagnosed with chronic renal failure and type 2 diabetes.

■ The short-term priority is to manage her diet to assist with achieving nutritional requirements and glycaemic control. Dietary approaches will assist with reducing risk of malnutrition and managing the biochemical effects of reduced renal function at the same time as maintaining control of weight and diabetic control. The dietary prescription may essentially consist of tailored amounts of protein, energy and fluid, together with control of sodium intake (and other nutrients according to clinical chemistry), all set, as far as possible, in the context of healthier eating (for diabetes control). The daily dietary prescription/intake would follow evidence-based guidelines, and consist of: energy 2100 kcal (35 kcal/kg) and a protein intake of about 40 g/d (36.1–42.1 g/d, based on a recommended intake of 0.6/0.7 g/d) with adequate monitoring to ensure the patient is not at risk of developing malnutrition. Fluid intake would normally be determined by fluid output (500 ml + previous 24-hr output). Sodium intake would normally be restricted to a NAS diet (80–100 mmol/d) to assist with blood pressure control. The patient would be advised to eat as healthily as possible in terms of fats (a lower fat intake with emphasis on unsaturated fatty acids) and carbohydrate (starchy foods at every meal) in the context of regular eating (frequent meals and snacks throughout the day). The prescription of energy, protein, fluid and sodium intake offered to the patient in the context of healthier eating, would jointly manage renal and diabetic clinical priorities.

■ In the longer term, priorities include securing optimal nutritional status in the midst of managing clinical control. Clinical chemistry suggests bone involvement (low calcium/high phosphate and alkaline phosphatase concentrations) and will require intervention (reducing exposure to dietary phosphorus, use of a phosphate binder, supplementation with active vitamin D, prevention of hypocalcaemia). Potassium levels should be checked and advice on formal restriction (avoidance of potassium-rich foods) may be necessary. Diet will be managed according to clinical chemistry and hence monitoring is essential. Avoidance of malnutrition is a longer-term priority and monitoring of weight and anthropometrical parameters will be important. Management of diabetes is also crucial and dietary review will be important to check compliance of all aspects of diet; of significance will be the consumption of a regular intake, containing fewer fat-containing foods and increased amounts of starch. Management of blood pressure and glycaemic control is crucial as this reduces the risk of development of microvascular disease, and may warrant tighter dietary sodium restriction. With reducing GFR over time, it will be important to review glycaemic control. If the patient is maintained on OHAs, then excretion of these drugs will be hampered and cause prolonged activity, resulting in greater hypoglycaemia risk (OHAs with long-term activity are hence contraindicated). A stricter management of carbohydrate intake may be useful here.

■ As the patient is reviewed (renal and diabetic services), the focus will be on clinical control of both renal and diabetic parameters. Weight monitoring is important and if weight is lost, this is putting the patient at nutritional risk. Thus, regular dietary review is essential, to provide information on why weight control may be jeopardised (e.g. appetite failure). Dietary advice will be informed by these data, and reinforcement of the aims of diet will be necessary, as appropriate.

■ As with any renal patient, the avoidance of malnutrition remains paramount as this is associated with poor clinical outcome. Monitoring over time is therefore crucial so that the necessary interventions can be put in place to ensure better treatment outcomes.

Case 55

■ There is evidence that nutritional status was good prior to the event. Nutritional requirements will be high and will be difficult to meet with a liquid diet. There may be challenges associated with eating/feeding, especially if the client is right-handed.

■ Assessment should consider the weight loss since the event (both pre- and post-operatively). It will be beneficial to consider this along with other measures of nutritional status (including % weight loss, rate of weight loss, ratio of fat mass : lean body mass and comparison of MAMC with reference rages). Use of waist circumference, as an alternative to BMI, may be appropriate. Assessment of diet (diet history and food intake records) and fluid intake (fluid balance charts) provides useful baseline information. Calculation of protein, fluid and energy requirements will provide the basis for the dietary intake. The client is clearly a good weight (and possibly quite muscular) and this should be taken into account in determining the intake. An accurate weight of the client (on the ward) is crucial to use in calculations. If this is not possible, then a usual weight prior to the event may suffice to calculate requirements, or perhaps using ideal body weight. The patient's weight may also be predicted using the clinical information given (BMI upper end of normal, height 6 ft 3 in = approximately 91 kg).

■ Calculations, based on a weight of 91 kg, may be assessed using predictive equations: Energy: BMR $15.1 \times 91 = 2066$ kcal; stress factor added of 10% (due to uncomplicated surgery) = 2273 kcal; add combined factor for activity and DIT (10%) = 2500 kcal/d. Protein: consider if protein stores are depleted resulting from trauma required for recovery, 0.2 g nitrogen (N) × 91 = 18.2 gN = 114 g protein/d. Fluid: consider evidence of pyrexia, no evidence in this patient, 35 ml × 91 = 3200 ml.

■ Practical considerations are important. The patient's appetite may be poor (due to pain, constipation and low mood) and may determine approaches. It may be important to look at hydration and biochemical status.

■ Short-term goals include trying to achieve nutritional requirements. A nutritional care plan should be negotiated with the client, nursing staff, care assistants and catering staff to ensure that a palatable, high energy/high protein liquid diet is provided to and is acceptable for, the patient. It is important to consider the likes and dislikes of the patient. The use of nutritional supplements, given the high level of requirements, may be considered if a fortified liquid diet does not meet requirements. The use of a high energy, nutritionally complete, supplement will provide maximum macro/micronutrient intake in a small volume. This may be preferable to presenting the patient with liquids requiring the use of wide-bore flexi-straws, which may be difficult to manage practically. A number of regimens are possible, to provide the aim of meeting nutritional requirements, an example of which is: a high energy/high protein liquid diet, fortified with milk powder, cream and sugar to provide 500 kcal/d and 35 g protein; a nutritionally complete (1.5 kcal/ml) milk-based liquid supplement to provide 2000 kcal/d and 74 g protein (e.g. 6 × 330 ml tetrapack).

■ If the patient is unlikely to meet requirements orally (e.g. if sedated), then consider supplementary nasogastric feeding overnight to provide 2000 kcal/d and 79 g protein.

■ In the longer term, nutritional goals include the priority of achieving and maintaining good nutritional status throughout treatment. The care plan should be reviewed weekly and changed as necessary. The patient should be reviewed prior to discharge, and suitable information discussed and negotiated with the client. The primary care dietitians should continue to review the patient.

Case 56

■ The short-term priorities must focus on meeting nutritional requirements, stabilising and then promoting weight gain. LBM must be preserved, and improved and pressure sore risk should be reduced. The diet should provide enough NSPs to promote regular bowel habit. Fluid status should be improved to promote and maintain good hydration. The diet should supply adequate vitamins and minerals to meet requirements to promote wound healing and reduce the risk of developing pressure sores.

■ At the six-month stage, the client is clearly not meeting nutritional requirements for energy and protein, and the formulation of reviewed and appropriate dietary advice is important and needs to be encouraged: appropriate/generous use of foods such as butter, milk and cheese, switch to small and frequent meal pattern, and to include puddings/desserts, the use of high energy snacks, such as creamy yoghurts and cake, the use of nourishing fluids (with or without thickener) such as full fat milk, use of appropriate texture of the diet; use of nutritional supplements (to include variety, taste preference) and how to incorporate these into the diet; the use of high energy supplements (powders) and how these can be added to foods.

■ Monitoring may include weight status, arm anthropometry and review of dietary intake (appetite and swallowing ability).

■ At the 18-month stage, calculation of the client's nutritional requirements forms the basis of the dietary intake, but method of feeding may include a gastrostomy feed to supplement oral intake (such as an overnight pump feed or bolus feeds during the day). Nutritionally complete (ready to hang) feeds or bolus sip feeds (using carton or unit) should be considered, and preference given to those with enhanced NSP content. Additional fluid can be given to meet requirements.

Case 57

■ Initial impressions strongly suggest that the client has some degree of liver impairment (raised ALT, bilirubin and alkaline phosphatase). The slightly raised ferritin level is also consistent with liver involvement. The client is overweight, but not diabetic (glucose levels within range) despite familial tendency. Consumption of alcohol is concerning (assume 750 ml of 12% wine, or higher) and may be interpreted to provide 18 units of ethanol in two days. This classifies the intake as binge drinking and will be detrimental to liver function (especially true of women); evidence at the present time suggests that alcohol consumption may be under-reported. If a fall in alcohol consumption is not anticipated, use of thiamine supplements may be indicated.

■ Reducing consumption of alcohol will assist in reduction of energy intake and have a beneficial impact on lipid profile. It would be useful to have baseline profiling information (HDL:LDL ratio) to act as a monitoring tool.

■ In the longer term, priorities include managing weight and lipid profiles to acceptable targets, involving the use of an energy-deficit, healthy eating diet plan containing optimal amounts of macronutrients. It may be useful to reduce sodium intake to recommended levels together with a reduction in saturated fat intake. Clearly, psycho-social factors linked to dietary and drinking behaviour may be set into goals in negotiation with the client. Consideration of lifestyle changes may be appropriate, such as physical activity.

■ Monitoring of weight, serum cholesterol, blood pressure, dietary changes and alcohol consumption will be useful. LFTs and blood pressure may be useful in clinical assessment.

Commentaries

Case 58

- Initial thoughts about this case are that the client may not be motivated (she refuses to be weighed) to comply with management of weight issues, and that weight (and shape) may be a psychological barrier for the patient.

- Initial assessment may begin with a food diary, which overcomes the need to ask the client lots of questions at the first interview. In many cases, a diary is a useful self-monitoring tool, as it raises awareness of what is actually eaten and drunk over a given period of time. The recording of information in the diary can often bring about change prior to the first encounter with the client, provided it is completed correctly (prospectively, and not at the end of each day, or every few days, i.e. retrospectively). Some clients bring a sanitised version, which is not helpful; some patients will not complete them because of the concerns they have about revealing their 'secret', or because of their literacy ability. Miss Ingram appears to be defensive, and may not want to divulge information about her eating behaviour.

- There are a number of areas to discuss at the first interview, in terms of short-term goals to improve positive behaviour and reduce energy intake including: shopping when not hungry, going to the local market to buy fruit and vegetables instead of visiting the supermarket (and succumbing to the tendency to shop more widely), shopping from a list (may curtail buying), only buying a couple of treats for the store cupboard, going to the petrol station only to buy petrol (could visit late at night when the shop inside is closed) and use of more appropriate snacks whilst watching television (or indeed finding a better use of her time). These changes in behaviour are what are perceived to make a difference, but the initial interview might concentrate on what the client wants to do, and therefore improve compliance.

- Together with the diary, it will be useful to assess the client with some cogent questions to determine: the stage of readiness to change on the behaviour change cycle (and discuss accordingly), the experience of trying to lose weight in the past (what was successful, and what was not) and her motivation (and compare this to previous diet experiences). The client should be assisted in making realistic goals (small dietary changes, weight loss and quality of diet), perhaps using an ambivalence grid or decisional balance to help her. It will be beneficial to identify some things that she wants to change and then ask her to prioritise her choices in terms of their importance and her confidence in carrying out the task(s) – if it is not important enough, or she is not confident, then she will likely fail.

- The intervention diet should be based on regular eating, healthy eating model, constructed using either 500 kcal/d energy deficit from baseline or calculated energy requirements (BMR + PAL). Merely giving up two chocolate bars will reduce her intake by this margin and induce some weight loss. The dietary intake, together with encouraging a modest exercise plan, can be monitored at clinic every 8–10 weeks or so, and the diet adjusted according to progress. Monitoring will be limited by her refusal to be weighed.

Case 59

- Initial thoughts about this case centre on the hospitalisation/home see-saw of relatively good and poor intakes. It may become increasingly difficult for the hospital to meet nutritional requirements since patients ultimately struggle to obtain adequate intakes from hospital diet. Unless nursed in single rooms, dietary intake may be hampered by the presence of other sick gastroenterology patients in ward situations and intakes are often negatively influenced by nil-by-mouth routines (medical tests).
- In the short term, the priority rests with achieving intake of energy and protein to meet requirements, and these may be calculated using predictive equations. The EAR for energy intake for healthy individuals in this age category is 1940 kcal. This client is almost certainly not consuming this. She is also likely to be physically inactive. Thus, achieving this level of intake may not be practical, but may be an ultimate target. The strategy must be: try oral hospital diet first (which may be supplemented with foods brought in from outside). If this does not satisfy requirements, then fortifying or supplementing foods may be the plan. Enteral feeding may be considered, with parenteral nutrition as a last resort.
- In the longer term, the priorities centre on achieving an appropriate weight which can be maintained consistently between hospital and home. Increasing calcium intake is appropriate to the level of 1500 mg/d (in view of steroid use and young female age category). Anaemia requires to be monitored (vitamin B_{12} and folate status). Smoking habit should be assessed as smoking is the single biggest environmental cause of flare-ups in Crohn's disease.
- This is a chronic condition and good rapport with the client is essential (probably across a MDT). A link with social workers may be useful, if there are problems at home. Monitoring issues include compliance with dietary instruction and maintaining a good intake of food when outwith the care setting.

Case 60

- Traditionally it was thought that milk caused diarrhoea and some doctors get confused and may actually ask a patient to avoid dairy products. In addition, undiagnosed coeliac disease may occur and should be excluded as a possibility. There has been some work done to link food intolerance with inflammatory bowel disease, but there is currently no evidence of a role for diet in the management of ulcerative colitis.
- On consideration of the blood test results, albumin concentration is low and it may be useful to see the WCC and CRP levels to ascertain whether the patient is malnourished or septic (the client is probably malnourished

on consideration of MAMC and TSF data). Haemoglobin and folate concentrations are also low and suggest anaemia; a diet/fluid history may reveal a poor intake of macro- and micronutrients (intake is probably low). Concentration of potassium is dangerously low and the cause needs to be ascertained; it may be potassium loss from the gastrointestinal tract, the patient may not be eating or there may be a gastrointestinal bleed (which needs to be corrected urgently). Sodium concentration is low, suggesting sodium depletion, but urinary electrolytes need to be checked to confirm or otherwise. It may be useful to check magnesium and vitamin D concentrations which may account for low levels of potassium. (In a patient with a high-output stoma, there may be huge gastrointestinal losses of magnesium. Low magnesium concentrations result in reduced secretion and function of PTH, further increasing renal losses of magnesium and indirectly reducing levels of 1,25 dihydroxyvitamin D.)

■ The objectives for dietary management are to improve his fluid and electrolyte balance (the main priority) and improve his nutritional status (to meet nutritional requirements more easily). The client needs to be educated about a better dietary and fluid intake.

■ Nutritional requirements for this client should be calculated using predictive formulae. Energy requirements, for a client aged 41 years: BMR (11.5 × 73) + 873 = 1713 kcal, and together with PAL (1.5 × 1713) = 2570 kcal/d. Protein requirements, for the same client: N = 0.2 × 73 = 14.6 gN = (× 6.25) = 91 g protein/d. The aim initially would be to establish a low fibre diet, restrict hypotonic fluids and offer sip feeds (polymeric), and double strength Dioralyte (1 litre/d).

■ Monitoring may include dietary intake (food record charts), MAMC and fluid balance (ensure output is reduced, and urinary output <1 litre/d). A priority for the client is to ensure that he understands that the more he drinks, the more his output will increase and the thirstier he will become. It may be useful to discuss the possibility that he may have bacterial overgrowth/pancreatic insufficiency or undiagnosed coeliac disease. If diarrhoea persists, then liaison with the pharmacist may be helpful (to ensure that loperamide and codeine are taken/or offered at appropriate times for the client).

Case 61

■ Initial impressions of this case suggest that the client will pose some difficulties. He is successful in business, and may be assertive, and clearly knows a lot about food. His weight may be impacting on his mobility problems. He comfort eats, and this may indicate other problems in his life, including work-related stress. Intervention would include some CBT with identification of his readiness to change. Initial targets should be negotiated with the client and preferably based on self-offered goals.

■ Waist measurement and BMI indicate strong risk for coronary heart disease and diabetes. Emphasis on reducing waist circumference may be preferable to focusing on his weight. Short-term goals should centre on establishing a regular meal pattern, and promoting consumption of a breakfast. Focus should clearly be on strategies to reduce comfort eating and nibbling food in the workplace. It is useful to engage the client with treatment, and getting him to target his nutritional knowledge by identifying dietary faults (intake of energy-dense foods and snacks, use of high fat/salty meats and alcohol) may assist in development of a personal plan. Involvement in light physical exercise will assist in managing weight loss and may provide distraction from eating, especially on his days off.

■ In the longer term, objectives will be to reinforce the link between poor diet behaviour (e.g. high salt intake and poor intake of nutrients) with existing (calcium and osteopenia) and potential (salt and blood pressure) problems, to help with motivation. Diet and lifestyle change should preferably be self-directed and negotiated. Diet changes should be in context – his access to Italian food need not centre on unhealthy food selection, but instead should favour more appropriate menu items, such as salads, fish, and alternative flavour sources, such as herbs and garlic. Stress relieving activities will assist in weight control (gentle exercise) and will help to reduce comfort eating.

■ The client needs to take more control of his dietary intake and lifestyle, and should engage with the concept of planning, rather than scavenging food that is easily accessible. Dietary advice must centre on healthy eating together with an energy deficit. A dietary history would assist in determining current food selection and portion sizes, with a view to planning a more appropriate intake. A suitable model of intervention may be based on the following energy deficit/requirements: BMR: $(11.6 \times 109) + 879\,kcal = 2143\,kcal/d$; PAL: $1.3 \times 2143 = 2786\,kcal/d$, to include a deficit (to induce weight loss) of 5–700 kcal = total energy intake of 2100–2300 kcal/d. The emphasis must be on reducing portion sizes, adopting a healthy eating approach to food and engaging in physical exercise. Ideas for food selection will be incorporated into dietary education materials for the client. A realistic pattern of weight loss may be discussed (perhaps 0.5–1.0 kg/week in the first instance) with reinforcement as achieving a target weight may take one to two years.

■ Monitoring may include weight checks, but perhaps monitoring waist circumference is more appropriate (to assess cardiovascular risk). The patient needs to agree a regular series of review appointments (perhaps every 10–12 weeks in the first instance) to monitor the extent to which dietary and lifestyle intervention is assisting weight control. Specific additional goals can be negotiated throughout the treatment period depending on progress.

Case 62

■ Initial impressions of the case are that the client was slightly overweight pre-pregnancy and is now obese (BMI $31\,kg/m^2$), following pre-conceptual dietary advice. The client needs to reduce her weight significantly to reduce the risk of developing diabetes. A GTT should have been performed to indicate a fasting blood glucose level <5.5 mmol/l (DMUK care recommendation). It may be useful to establish if she is planning the children's dietary intakes and snacking on foods rejected by them and indeed whether she is preparing healthy meals for them (she is gaining weight and this is not clear).

■ Initial assessment suggests that there is a strong motivational factor in the family history of diabetes. The client needs encouragement to take the time to consider herself more and may benefit from taking more physical exercise (the puppy is unlikely to generate much exercise, although may influence spare time activities).

■ Short-term nutritional goals should stress the need to plan her own dietary intake more, as opposed to scavenging foods rejected by the children. Preparing and cooking healthy foods suitable for both the client and her children requires reinforcement (can modify consistency according to stage of weaning). The client may benefit from increased cardiovascular activity and reinforcement of the understanding of a healthy diet. Assessment of her current intake of energy-dense foods may assist in diet planning.

■ Dietary intervention may be based on estimation of energy requirements to induce weight loss and may be based on a predictive equation: BMR = (8.3 × 97.5) + 846 = 1655 kcal; PAL = 1655 × 1.5 = 2482 kcal (assuming moderately active). To assist weight reduction, an energy deficit of 500 kcal may be applied to the diet plan = 2482 − 500 = 1982 kcal or approximately 2000 kcal/d. This energy prescription may then be woven into a healthy eating diet plan and the client instructed using motivational approaches to encourage behaviour modification. The current diet may be assessed to establish preferred foods and the client educated.

■ In the longer term, reinforcement of the impact of diet on cholesterol levels and hypertension and diabetes risk would be helpful. In addition, reinforcement of healthy eating messages and advice given previously would assist with compliance. Longer-term goal setting needs to be adjusted as short-term achievements are made.

■ Monitoring and evaluation may include weight checks (four weekly) and dietary review (dietary history and recall). Food diaries may be useful as a self-monitoring tool prior to reviews. Blood pressure and routine blood lipid screen would assist in monitoring cardiovascular risk (started three months from baseline).

■ Particular challenges presented by this case include the difficulty of managing changes to diet and lifestyle without help and support at home (partner, family and friends).

Case 63

■ On admission, the patient has a BMI of 27 kg/m² and his nutritional requirements may be calculated using predictive equations. Energy requirements may be assessed using BMR = (11.4 × 83) + 870 = 1816 kcal, with a further 10% (immobility), 10% for stress (fracture) and 40% for ventilation = a daily energy requirement of 2900 kcal. Protein requirements may be calculated using $0.17-0.20 \text{gN} \times 83 = 14.1-16.6 \text{gN/d} = 88-104 \text{g}$ protein/d. Fluid requirements $= 35 \text{ml} \times 83 = 2900 \text{ml/d}$. The gut is functioning, therefore a nasogastric feed is appropriate. The patient should be fed in the short term, with a need for review (ventilation and sedation, nil-by-mouth).

- ▪ Short-term goals include meeting his nutritional and fluid requirements. There is a need to consider medication to treat seizures (if phenytoin is being given, breaks in feeding may be required). Maintenance of weight and promotion of wound healing (facial laceration and fracture) are also priorities. Monitoring includes ensuring that the patient is receiving the feed prescribed. The patient's weight should be reviewed if the patient comes off the ventilator; otherwise, arm anthropometric assessment should be conducted at initial and review visits to patient to monitor changes in fat and muscle stores. Assessment of fluid balance (especially output) is important, as is monitoring of urine and blood electrolytes.

- ▪ Estimated nutritional requirements need to be reviewed (especially at day 10), as ventilation is discontinued and the stress factor may be deleted from the calculation. If the patient is too sleepy to walk, but is sitting up, then an activity factor may be added (15%). Oral intake should be assessed: if the patient is able to eat, then liaison with the SLT is important (for a swallow assessment). If the patient is unable to eat orally, or has an unsafe swallow assessment, then continue nasogastric feeding (hydration, and to meet full requirements).

- ▪ At day 14, the SLT requires to complete a swallow assessment and when eating commences, a food record chart should form part of daily observations. The intake records should inform progress; food and drink intake should be reviewed and nutritional requirements reassessed periodically. The patient should be advised of menu options and should be given guidance as to appropriate food choices. Oral diet, together with supplements may be appropriate (to meet requirements); nasogastric feeding may be continued/adjusted according to how much oral diet is tolerated. The aim will be to reduce feed gradually as oral diet increases. Weight should be monitored, together with food intake records. Account should be taken of the SLT's notes and information concerning wound healing. When full oral feeding is established, and the patient is meeting nutritional requirements with hospital diet, oral supplements should be discontinued.

Case 64

- ▪ Initial impressions suggest a client who values a good quality of life and key points include significant weight loss, reduction of appetite and at risk of malnutrition. Planned treatments may impact further on nutritional intake and if treatment is delivered in different centres, transfer of information may be crucial in maintaining standards of care. There may be local or national support group information available.

- Assessment may include calculation of his BMI ($21.07 \, kg/m^2$ – normal range), assessment of weight lost (6.4 kg) and percentage weight loss (8.6% in three months; at risk of malnutrition) and consideration of his low albumin concentration (which may be disease-specific rather than an indicator of nutritional status).
- Short-term nutritional/dietary and lifestyle goals may include: optimising nutritional intake (given the progressive dysphagia), arranging follow-up reviews within a set time frame, coordinating care around planned dates for treatment, ensuring goals are patient-focused (discussing and negotiating options rather than being prescriptive) and ensuring that information given is supported by other health professionals involved in the client's care.
- In the longer term, goals may be to optimise nutritional intake given the treatment side-effects and surgical intervention, give post-operative advice in a timely manner and ensure this is understood, offer follow-up reviews within a set time frame and consider the client returning to 'normal' diet as a clinical outcome after completion of treatment. Consultation and advice should be discussed with carers, as well as the patient.
- Dietary and nutrition interventions may be planned following formal assessment of dietary intake. This may include advice on fortification of food and texture modification which needs to be individualised, documented, written in patient-friendly format and verbally reinforced. The use of supplements may be considered, exploring issues of taste fatigue, mixing into food, any new products that may be available and the cost to the primary care service. The client may require enteral tube feeding which needs to be fully explained. The client needs reassurance if the dietary intake does not meet expectations or requirements as the treatment side-effects may have a significant effect on intake. Liaison with the multi-professional team with regard to symptom control is important (post-chemotherapy).
- Weight may be monitored and post-operative weight differences from baseline noted. Clinical chemistry and anthropometry may be appropriate, subject to patient consent (MAMC and TST). Liaison with service in primary care may be appropriate given length of time until follow-up; information transfer is important.
- Care complications in this case are presented by progressive dysphagia and in planning treatment over a long time frame between hospital and primary care service. Ensure follow-up is available and of a consistent level of expertise. The client may also have consulted with the Internet for information on complementary therapy/alternative diets.

Case 65

- The case presents a few complex issues: the client is a long-standing diabetic and will have pre-conceived ideas about his management (a health professional). In addition, he has no immediate family support.

- Short-term goals include tackling the total energy intake, in addition to intake of protein and fat. Because of immobility following a fall his energy intake should be decreased, and to perhaps about 1900 kcal/d. His total fat intake also needs to fall; this will partly be addressed by a reduction in energy intake and reducing his heavy reliance on intake of convenience foods (often energy-dense and containing little else but fat and sugar). The client needs a dietary review followed by advice centring on a suitable meal structure with regular balanced meals that contain more low glycaemic index (and fresh) foods and intake of more modest portions.

- His long-term diabetic control is poor, despite being on short-acting insulin. It may be worth considering establishment of a background insulin (such as Lantus or Levemir) to even out his control, and thus reduce doses of short-acting insulin. Consideration may also be given to the use of metformin to assist with control in spite of insulin resistance and to assist weight management. UKPDS and DCCT state the importance of balancing the diet to minimise risk of complications – it may be useful to strengthen advice to the client using this information. Blood pressure requires tighter control; salt restriction can be partly targeted to reinforce this issue, and the case for reduction in intake of convenience foods. Modest physical exercise should be encouraged as part of lifestyle modification.

- It may be appropriate to monitor this patient fairly frequently to begin with (monthly) to assess weight, diet/micronutrient balance, glycaemic control and blood pressure. Evaluation may take the form of home blood glucose monitoring; his readings do not conform with HbA_{1c} assessment or weight history.

- This case presents the difficulty of an independent client who may lack even basic cooking skills. It may be useful to encourage him to enrol on a healthy eating cooking course to increase confidence in adequately managing his own diet, together with improving glycaemic control, weight control and blood pressure to minimise the risk of complications. Visits to the Orient Express may continue, but could be viewed more as a treat, than as a regular feature of the client's diet. The client may be resistant to increasing physical activity; he might consider an intensive scheme (12 weeks) which might also incorporate healthy eating and encourage him to make social contact with others.

Case 66

- The case presents a young married man, adjusting to a new life in a different culture. He is overweight/obese (with a waist circumference of 98 cm) with modestly elevated blood pressure. His dietary intake may be assisting both to his tendency to obesity (high fat/high energy intake) and high blood pressure (high salt intake). There is clearly a need to establish a healthier eating pattern, whist retaining a traditional Polish diet. Any language barrier may require the use of an interpreter or English-speaking member of the family.

Commentaries

■ Assessment of the client may involve a full dietary history to identify any dietary weaknesses. Particular inspection of dietary fat and sodium intake may form the particular approach in guiding the formation of a suitable intervention diet. The client appears to be quite active, but a lifestyle assessment may be useful (e.g. amount of exercise and alcohol consumption). Clearly the dietitian may need to become familiar with dietary components of a traditional Polish intake and should visit the Polish centre of the city.

■ Short-term dietary priorities include reducing exposure to high fat and salty foods. This may be best achieved by reducing portion sizes of traditionally eaten foods (especially processed meats and fish products), rather than exclusion of these familiar foods (and incurring compliance issues). The extent to which the client may move away from traditional foods, towards a healthier intake may be a good starting point for an initial consultation. Reducing exposure to alcoholic beverages may also be a priority (based on actual consumption).

■ In the longer term, priorities may include management of weight, although this may form part of the initial consultation. An accurate assessment of energy intake may be helpful in forming an appropriate intervention diet, based on a healthy eating, energy-deficit model. This would be based on a calculation of BMR, together with a factor for activity (may be light or moderate, depending on lifestyle assessment) and inclusion of an energy-deficit factor of the order of 5–700 kcal/d. The diet would be planned incorporating as many traditional foods as possible, paying particular attention to reduce intake of high fat/high sodium foods (blood sausages and pork crackling) and capitalising on more appropriate foods (vegetables and pickles). It may be that some dietary components are very concentrated sources of salt, and these should be avoided.

■ Monitoring of blood pressure and dietary changes would form the main ongoing assessments and may fall to the practice dietitian and nurse. Waist circumference may be the most practical tool to monitor weight management. Assessment of compliance with the diet may be the focus of a dietary review. Follow-up assessments may be eight to ten weekly or through arrangements made with the occupational health department.

Commentaries

Case 67

■ This is a case of a young man who will require to make significant behaviour modification, but has questionable motivation. It is not clear who has requested dietary advice, but we could assume that a meeting between the client and the family doctor has taken place. Poor diet does not appear to be the main problem; focus should perhaps be on managing the depression. There are signs of increasing activity levels (swimming). Impression of the diet suggests that it may not be overly high in fat, sugar or salt content, but there is clearly room for improvement in the shape of increasing intake of cardio-protective foods and including more dietary variety. He may need emotional support (counselling or specialist input) to try to reduce dependency on medications (e.g. anti-depressants). There is a need to find out what may be meant by long-term health issues so that a practical and realistic treatment plan and appropriate support can be arranged from the primary care MDT. The need for signposting may come up during the initial consultation: to appropriate local services for support to return to work and to appropriate local rehabilitation support/smoking cessation services (use of recreational drugs and cigarettes). Medications may be contributing to problems: more detail about stabilising drug use would help.

■ Assessment of the case includes noting his blood pressure, which may put him at high risk of cardiovascular disease, and may be caused by sodium intake in association with stress/anxiety. His BMI indicates overweight, which is a health risk (however, only 5% weight loss would be required to reach normal BMI; aim for 6.5 kg total weight loss). Waist circumference measurement would be useful to confirm cardiovascular risk and act as a monitoring tool. Initial impressions of his diary suggest an average intake of sodium and energy content in comparison with usual UK intakes. Daily dietary intake is estimated to contain (using average portions and averaged across the days): 1970 mg sodium (4.9 g salt) and energy (1830 kcal). The client's salt intake is therefore lower than usual UK intakes (9.5 g) and falls within the recommended maximum intake of 6 g salt/d. (Salt intake was based on assumptions: tuna in oil, salted butter and that salt was not added to cooking.) Estimated average requirements for energy, based on his age and activity level of 1.4, are 2550 kcal/d. The client's intake is less than this; his activity level may be lower than 1.4. There is no evidence of an alcohol intake exceeding recommendations, but alcohol may contribute significant amounts of energy. Intake of fruit and vegetables is likely to be lower than recommended. Intakes of omega-3 fats, MUFA, oily fish and NSP are poor.

■ Dietary and lifestyle goals include: achieving ideal body weight (reduce by 6.5 kg over time) which will assist with blood pressure control and reduce cardiovascular risk and risk of developing the metabolic syndrome. Increasing physical activity to recommended levels of duration, together with incorporating relaxation, may be useful. Maintaining a low intake of salt (positive dietary reinforcement/education) through use of freshly prepared foods is a priority; the client can be taught how to read food labels and to use alternative flavouring agents. Increasing intake of fruit and vegetables is also a priority; adoption of the Mediterranean-style diet will assist in achieving an intake of four to six portions of fruit and two to three portion of vegetables/d. Increasing intake of cardio-protective foods (three to four portions oily fish/week and omega-3 fatty acid-containing foods) is wise (or consider using an omega-3 fatty acid supplement). The diet may be presented to the client using a healthy eating model, including advice about safe levels of alcohol intake and how to meet energy requirements.

Commentaries

■ In the longer term, goals include maintenance of normal weight and support of continuation with lifestyle changes. Follow-up arrangements may include liaison with any support agencies involved to determine outstanding issues affecting morale and motivation of the client. Waist circumference may be useful to monitor health risk (as opposed to weight parameters). It may be useful to monitor the client every four to six weeks over a six-month period and then discharge to the practice nurse and GP for ongoing monitoring and care.

Case 68

■ Significant points of the case indicate that nutritional screening needs to be done on admission and weekly whilst an in-patient together with monitoring weekly (and notably weight). The aim is to meet nutritional requirements; if the patient is only on liquid diet, then there may be a need to consider nutrition support (nasogastric feeding or use of nutritional supplements). Oral intake should be monitored and appropriate nutritional support considered as the patient progresses from liquids to hospital diet. There may be a need to consider use of high-energy snacks or supplements. The meals provided should be of a suitable texture (e.g. puréed, soft). Monitoring of weight, dietary (food records) and fluid intake is important, together with urine and clinical chemistry (electrolytes). Assistance will need to be provided for eating and drinking to support intake; input from a SLT would be ideal and useful from the outset (swallow assessment). Similarly, involvement of the MDT will be useful from the start of care (e.g. physiotherapist, occupational therapist).
■ Short-term goals include the priority of meeting nutritional and fluid requirements and implies adequate monitoring of oral intake (diet records/history) and indicates level and nature of nutritional support. There is a need for regular dietary review. Target weight parameters should be maintained (and monitored at least weekly). The patient needs to be kept adequately hydrated (and fluid balance monitored, together with urine metabolites and blood electrolytes). Risk of development of pressure sores will be reduced if the patient is meeting requirements. There is a need to provide adequate textured nutrition as the patient progresses and the SLT requires to review the client regularly.
■ The longer-term goals centre on maintaining nutritional and fluid status. There is still a need to monitor weight parameters and the aim is to eat a full hospital diet; it may be useful to advise the client on healthier options from the hospital menu. The need to assist the patient to eat needs to be reviewed and given when necessary. Ultimately the aim will be to encourage intake of a balanced diet and provide advice for home discharge on healthy eating, reducing salt intake and consuming a minimum of five portions of fruit and vegetables/d. Lipid profile can be checked, and advice on how to follow a cardio-protective diet given.

▪ Discharge objectives centre on the above information; advice on modified diet texture will form the nature of dietary advice. Dietetic review once home is important. The patient is obese and therefore advice on reducing weight is important (balanced, probably energy-deficit healthy eating dietary advice). It will be useful to have a discharge weight to benchmark future weight information. It may be useful to liaise with the SLT for discharge care. Home circumstances require consideration and advice planned accordingly (e.g. presence of family support). The patient should be discharged with diet priorities and referred to the community rehabilitation team. If there are raised lipid levels on discharge, these need to be followed up (every 10–12 weeks), and dietary advice tailored to reduce these.

▪ If a PEG feeding tube is used, additional information needs to be given concerning care for a clean, healthy stoma site. Monitoring may be more frequent (daily fluid balance, weekly urine and electrolyte status) and the oral intake reviewed weekly. When discharged, the patient will manage daily PEG maintenance and care, and the monitoring should continue, but move to four- to eight-weekly review. Calculation of new nutritional requirements will be necessary and the diet planned accordingly. Bowel habit must be reviewed to avoid constipation, and the diet planned accordingly.

Case 69

▪ Initial impressions of the case suggest that the patient is normally fit and well with a presumed good food intake. This view is supported by a normal-to-healthy BMI ($24\,kg/m^2$). However, the patient has been left for >72 hr prior to feeding which is not in accordance with national guidelines for management of stroke victims.

▪ Baseline assessment: all serum levels are within normal ranges on admission, but all at the higher end of normal. This is likely to reflect some underlying dehydration caused by the patient being without fluids for up to 16 hours prior to admission. This will be quickly corrected on administration of intra-venous fluids. CRP and albumin levels are normal, indicating that there is no underlying infection. Interpretation of these results would be assisted by fluid balance information and clinical observation of skin turgor.

▪ Some blood tests would assist in determining the feeding regimen, including plasma/serum urea, electrolytes, magnesium, phosphorus and corrected calcium (re-feeding syndrome may be likely now that the patient has been five days nil-by-mouth). Levels of these nutrients need to be corrected as required.

▪ The regimen needs to be constructed to meet nutritional requirements. Fluid balance needs to be monitored to identify under/over hydration and allow amendment in the fluid provided. Monitoring of urine and blood electrolytes, serum/plasma magnesium, corrected calcium and phosphorus should continue after feeding and then two to three times a week or more frequently if levels are abnormal and requiring correction. Abdominal function should be monitored (nausea, vomiting and bowel movement). There is a need to confirm the position of the naso-gastric tube with pH indicator paper (and a pH <5.5 prior to use of tube).

■ Requirements should be calculated using predictive equations. Energy: BMR = $(9.8 \times 62) + 624 = 1232$ kcal, addition of a stress factor = +5% (62kcal) = 1294 kcal, and addition of activity factor = +15% (185 kcal) = 1479 kcal/d. Protein = $0.17 \times 62 = 10.54$ gN = 66g protein/d. Fluid requirement = $30 \times 62 = 1860$ ml.

■ An appropriate feeding regimen may be:
Day 1: Jevity 50 ml/hr × 20 hr, continue with 24-hr intra-venous fluids (i.e. 1000 ml) (= 1000 kcal, 40 g protein, 2000 ml).
Day 2: Jevity 75 ml/hr × 20 hr, water 100 ml/hr × 4 hr (= 1500 kcal, 60 g protein, 1900 ml).
Day 3: Jevity 100 ml/hr × 15 hr, water 150 ml/hr × 2 hr (= 1500 kcal, 60 g protein, 1500 ml).

Case 70

■ Initial impressions of this case indicate a palliative care patient for whom optimising nutritional intake in relation to quality of life is a priority.

■ This case is difficult to solve due to the limited information provided (size of tumour, effects on gastrointestinal function including bowel or oesophagus involvement/obstruction, or whether any palliative intervention has been established, such as placing of a stent). The assumption is that the patient is at end stage if requiring hospice admission.

■ Short-term goals include trying to stabilise weight and dietary intake. With a BMI of 17 kg/m², and a 19% weight loss (over three months), this is clinically significant and indicates use of nutritional support. It will be crucial to identify current intake and any physical effects the tumour may have in influencing dietary intake. This would allow the dietitian to make the distinction between weight loss being caused by the tumour or due to the reduced intake. The plan would probably be to aim for small, frequent meals that are energy-dense and protein rich, and may include the use of standard nutritional supplements. Cancer-specific supplements (enriched with EPA) may be indicated where weight loss occurs despite a good food intake and the tumour is appropriate for intervention. In hospital, use of a high protein/energy-dense menu will provide suitable food, drink and snacks.

■ Ideally the patient should be seen pre-operatively because of low BMI and weight loss. Clinical guidelines recommend the use of outpatient screening and the need for inpatient screening to be completed within 24 hours of admission. In this case, weight loss and muscle wasting reduce the overall effect on quality of life and may compromise clinical outcomes.

Commentaries

■ Requirements should be calculated, using standard predictive equations. Energy: BMR $= (11.5 \times 52) + 873 = 1471$ kcal, with the addition of a stress factor of 5% (+74 kcal) and with the addition of an activity factor of 15% (+221 kcal) $= 1765$ kcal/d (+500 kcal). Protein: $0.17 \times 52 = 8.84$ gN $= 55$ g protein/d. Fluid requirement $= 35 \times 52 = 2170$ ml. If the general hospital diet is taken in full amounts, then requirements will be met, but it is likely that only partial amounts will be taken. Thus, fortified foods and the use of energy-dense snacks is indicated. It is likely that additional supplements will be required to meet requirements in conjunction with an acceptable diet to the patient.

■ It is crucial to determine exactly how 'end-stage' the patient is; putting emphasis on meeting requirements and promoting weight gain may not be prudent in a patient in the very end stages. Approach with a very ill patient should focus on the positives of small goals of increasing dietary intake. Monitoring weight may also not be a priority in a very ill patient; further weight loss may have a negative effect on the patient. Consideration of more aggressive feeding will depend on stage in relation to palliative use of chemo/radiotherapy. Monitoring and regular follow-up and assessment of intake and compliance with uptake of diet, snacks, or feeds will be useful. Written information regarding the desired and managed intake of the patient should be part of the transfer arrangement from hospital to hospice. Ensuring prescription of supplements is crucial.

Commentaries

The commentaries: the diaries

Consideration of the diaries reveals the following observations and may help inform appropriate dietary, nutritional and lifestyle approaches and advice.

Diary 1

- Eating pattern is relatively regular and frequent.
- There is a disparity in dietary intake between days (Edinburgh/home intakes are associated with meal planning, resulting in a better qualitative intake; Glasgow/'away' intakes are associated with reduced access to preferred foods and the client must resort to consuming foods generally accepted to be less healthy).
- Dietary restraint is associated with Edinburgh days (note food selection and quantities); greater dietary freedom is associated with Glasgow days (note food selection).
- Edinburgh days are unlikely to meet energy requirements; Glasgow days are more likely to meet energy requirements, but quality of intake may be compromised (intake of saturated fat, sodium).
- Assigning the cause of weight loss is problematic and may be partly attributed to dietary restraint on more of the days, exercise and training and the presence of a worm.
- Treatment of anaemia, or eradicating the worm (removing the cause) will generally improve dietary intake.
- Dietary intake may benefit from trying to align diet with a healthy eating model and may include improving intake of NSPs and achieving optimal dietary intakes of protein, energy and fluid, and perhaps making more informed food choices on Glasgow days.

Diary 2

- Eating pattern is relatively regular and frequent.
- The dietary intake is relatively healthy, compared with a healthy eating dietary model, except for the intake of chocolate and chocolate-containing snack foods.
- Likely dietary triggers for headache include chocolate, caffeine and wine. Dietary intake of these may be significant.
- The client scavenges for food and eats rejected or left-over food from the baby.
- Advice may centre on keeping the general shape of the diet (healthy foods) and maintaining good intakes of nutrients to support development of maternal and fetal growth.
- The client should eliminate dietary triggers, at least for a trial period (wine and chocolate), and note any change in headache severity or pattern.

- The client may be advised to plan her intake and thus avoid scavenging on left-overs and perhaps inappropriate foods.
- Dietary intake may benefit from increasing fluid intake to recommended levels with appropriate fluids (advice on caffeine-free beverages).

Diary 3

- Eating pattern is relatively regular and frequent.
- Dietary intake shows evidence of dietary restraint, including intake of skimmed milk, low calorie beverages and lower fat cooking methods.
- Dietary intake compares quite well with a healthy eating model of intake.
- Weighed portion/serving sizes show commitment to a regulated approach to intake, although some serving sizes may need adjustment.
- It may be appropriate to centre the advice on keeping the broad shape of her diet as it is, but perhaps focusing on improvement of intake of NSP and consistent levels of fluid intake (to meet recommendations for health), together with increasing physical activity to recommended levels.
- Omission of inappropriate dietary items may be appropriate (e.g. cheese scone, sponge cake).
- It may be appropriate to assess energy intake/output and formulate and reinforce modest weight loss/physical activity advice.

Diary 4

- Eating pattern is relatively regular and frequent, but snacking behaviour predominates.
- Quantitative inspection of the diet suggests that large portion/serving sizes of inappropriate foods may be predominating.
- Qualitative dietary intake suggests a higher than advisable intake of fat, sodium and alcohol (Sunday) to meet general health principles and perhaps coincides with symptomatology.
- Late eating and reliance on convenience foods may not be conducive to optimal bowel function and habit and will almost certainly result in epigastric pain (dyspepsia) and symptom development later in the day.
- Dietary approaches may take the form of trying to align her diet with a healthy eating model, focusing on reducing intake of snack foods and increasing intake of fresh and cooked foods in the form of meals. Food selection should centre on containing less fat and sodium; meal frequency, especially later in the evening, should be reduced. The client may benefit from modifying intake of alcohol and taking regular exercise.
- The client has reported in her history that she associates intake of bread, pasta and dairy foods with symptoms. If a healthy eating approach does not assist with reduction in severity of symptoms, it may be useful to attempt to reduce the client's exposure to wheat, and/or dairy foods for

a prescribed period of time to assess the potential of these two food groups to ameliorate symptoms.

Diary 5

- Eating pattern is relatively regular and frequent, with the classic and traditional dietary intake of three meals and three snacks.
- Diet diaries are meticulously recorded (amounts in grams), perhaps indicating an exceptional interest and pre-occupation with diet and related issues (also, she sent the diary *ahead* of the consultation).
- Inclusion of the information about dietary supplements gives further evidence of the client's concern about her dietary intake. Indeed, the nature of the supplements chosen, and reliance on these, may suggest obsession with her health and general health issues.
- Familial disease may result in undue interest in health; the consultant may have inadvertently heightened the client's desire to reduce serum cholesterol levels to an unrealistic clinical outcome.
- Prescription of statin drugs suggests a greater level of clinical control is required (familial hypercholesterolaemia).
- Self-prescription of supplements indicates a desire to assist clinical control, regardless of the evidence on which they are based, and suggests a controlled client with a very prescriptive outlook on life.
- The nutritional quality of the intake is likely to be very close to an ideal intake to reduce cardiovascular risk, but strongly suggestive of an intake that is impractical for most individuals.
- The approach taken at interview might well tackle the impractical measures taken by this client, but it is important not to stifle motivation. Reducing the client's reliance on dietary supplements may not be unreasonable, but again, this may need to be handled with care.
- It may be useful to consider other lifestyle approaches to reduction of serum cholesterol, such as modest, sustained physical activity.

Diary 6

- Eating pattern is relatively regular and frequent.
- Quantitatively, his serving/portion sizes are large, especially of meat, bread and snack foods.
- Qualitatively, the client's dietary variety is good, but there is obvious preference for meat, convenience foods, salty foods and thus his diet is likely to contain high amounts of protein, fat and sodium. Intake of sweet foods, and therefore of simple carbohydrates is likely to be high. Intake of dietary energy is high, in view of consumption of so many energy-dense foods. Intake of complex carbohydrates is low.
- Since kidney stones and gout are more likely to occur in individuals consuming large amounts of protein from animal sources (meat), it is likely that the client's current diet constitutes significant risk of stone formation.

Commentaries

- Since the client's intake contains large amounts of fat and salt, it is likely the diet represents considerable risk for hypertension.
- Since the client's dietary intake comprises so many energy-dense foods, and is therefore likely to exceed energy requirements, the intake is likely to assist with weight gain and therefore increase hypertension risk.
- The diet plan and approach for Mr Redpath would centre on reducing energy intake, especially reducing exposure to dietary fat and protein (to normal percentage energy partition), together with switching to fresh sources of meat (to reduce sodium intake) and fish, which are grilled or roasted, instead of fried. In addition, reducing obvious sources of fat (cream, butter, fried foods and cheese) would help to bring the general shape of the diet into line with optimum percentages of macronutrient intake. Increasing the dietary intake of NSPs and appropriate fluids would assist with diluting urine (and hence reduce stone formation risk) and improving the spread of nutrition. Limiting intake of snack foods and switching to lower energy drinks ('diet drinks') would assist with weight control.
- It is likely that reducing serving sizes represents a difficulty, since Australians are good meat eaters and may be resistant to changing to smaller portions.
- Increasing physical exercise and general mobility, together with reducing exposure to alcohol, may also be priorities for lifestyle improvement.

Diary 7

- Eating pattern is relatively regular and very frequent.
- Quantitatively, serving/portion sizes are likely to be normal.
- Qualitatively, there is a reasonable spread of nutrition, in terms of macronutrients, and the load of fat and protein is unlikely to be excessive. However, there is a tendency to consume high intakes of simple carbohydrates and symptoms of light-headedness appear to be connected with this feature of the client's intake.
- Ideally, the plan and approach may be to reduce dietary exposure to simple sugars and increase intake of wholegrain cereals in an attempt to avoid the risk of reactive hypoglycaemia.
- Practical suggestions for snack foods high in NSPs and low in simple sugars may be beneficial for the client.
- It may also be useful to roughly gauge whether the current dietary intake meets the energy requirements of a physically active young woman.
- Re-assessment of symptom development would prove useful at a review appointment in response to the 'new' diet.
- The reason for self-limiting dietary intake of pasta and bread may be due to either a self-belief that these may effect control of weight or may be influencing development of symptoms. It will be useful to explore these issues at the interview.

Diary 8

- Eating pattern is relatively regular and frequent.
- There is evidence of reducing dietary exposure to both dairy and wheat components of her diet.
- Over-emphasis on a restricted diet may compromise energy intake, as may be the case here. It may be useful to scan the intakes to inform a crude judgement of energy intake. There is also evidence of general dietary restraint (low fat houmous, 'slim-line' tonic).
- Submission of four weeks of diet diaries may be significant – the client may be exhibiting signs of over-interest in her diet (this is also true of her interest in the Internet to trial new diets).
- The dietary plan may be to align the dietary intake, as far as possible, with a healthy eating model, and ascertain whether the client is happy to continue with a dairy-free, wheat-free dietary regimen, as there appears to be little justification for this medically.
- The 'new' diet should conform with the client's preferences, and should ensure an intake of plenty of fluids (to combat effects of dehydration resulting from diarrhoea).
- It may be useful to consider intakes of NSPs – is the client eating enough insoluble carbohydrate?
- There is evidence of the client worrying about her intake and being over-pre-occupied with her intake – this may be causing undue stress, and exacerbation of the diarrhoea. It may be useful to ascertain whether other stresses may be influencing bowel habit, and perhaps examine the possibility of increasing physical exercise.

Diary 9

- Eating pattern is relatively regular and frequent but there is a preference for snacking behaviour.
- Quantitatively, portion/serving sizes are not given, and therefore assumptions only may be made about quantities of foods/drinks consumed.
- Qualitatively, the diet is probably high in fat, sugar and alcohol, and probably low in NSPs and the nutrients supplied by both soluble and insoluble carbohydrates.
- It is difficult to gauge the energy supplied by the dietary intake based on these dietary records, but it may be that it does not supply enough energy (resulting in night hunger and the need to get up in search of food).
- The diet plan would be to assess intake of NSPs and fluid and align the diet with a healthy eating model of intake.
- In addition, physical activity may be explored, in terms of training, and the energy and fluid (and possibly protein) requirements calculated, and the new diet calibrated to include sensible levels of these nutrients.

Commentaries

Diary 10

- Eating pattern is relatively erratic, in terms of timing, and reflects lifestyle commitments across both days.
- The client has submitted diaries for 14 days. This may suggest either an eagerness to demonstrate appropriate eating patterns or a real desire to treat weight loss seriously.
- The dietary intake clearly represents a variety of food and drink intake together with a reasonable intake of healthy food with obvious exceptions (turkey pieces, deep fried, but home-made).
- For a client who has dabbled with different diets to assist with losing weight, significantly a high protein, high fat, low carbohydrate diet often results in a difficulty to manage with smaller portions of meat or fish. It is not clear from the diary here, but may be clarified at interview.
- The client may well be either motivated or demoralised, by the impact of various family members who may be classified as athletes, and therefore successful in their various events.
- Clearly, dietary intakes and patterns are better at the weekends, and part of any approach may be to try to bring regular eating patterns closer to these (these are associated with differences in lifestyle). Work appears to be stressful, and associated with a poorer dietary intake. Access to healthier foods may also be hampered and restricted to what is available at work.
- The approach taken may be to align the diet with a healthy eating model of intake and avoid obvious food items that are energy-dense.
- Nutritional goals should be set, both in the short and longer term, which may include weight projections. However, aggressive weight loss is not part of the plan, and the client needs to be aware of the need to lose weight gradually and strategically. Setting realistic targets and monitoring these over an appropriate time frame is appropriate.

The commentaries: the referrals

Consideration of the patient/client referrals reveals the following observations and may help inform appropriate dietary, nutritional and lifestyle approaches and advice.

Referral 1

- The client is clearly motivated and will most likely benefit from appropriate cardioprotective dietary advice (implementation of a Mediterranean-style diet, and replacement of saturated fats with unsaturated fats), rather than lipid-lowering advice *per se*. It may be that she has a healthy diet and needs reassurance that she is already eating appropriately. Alternatively, her diet may benefit from 'fine tuning'.
- Assessment of the case indicates that she has a history of raised total and LDL cholesterol levels as statin treatment was required. The consultant physician may feel she would gain additional benefit from even lower levels of LDL, perhaps because of the significant risk attributed to factors such as smoking, family history and raised blood pressure (she is relatively young). The client will benefit from reassurance that increasing the dose of statins is likely to optimise LDL lowering and that there is a need to focus on a cardioprotective diet. Exercise will boost HDL level and reduce CHD progression, and lifestyle advice is clearly important. If she is a smoker, advice must be given to stop smoking. If she consumes alcohol, then this must be within target recommendation.
- In the short term, goals will be to encourage the client to continue with any recent self-implemented changes, such as dietary improvement, cessation of smoking, moderation of alcohol intake and increasing physical activity. Approaches taken should be reassuring. Focus should then concentrate on further dietary improvement, such as reducing intake of SFA and switching to increased amounts of unsaturated fatty acids, increasing fruit and vegetable consumption to at least five portions a day, limiting intake of sugar and salt intake and consuming more oily fish. One to two dietary goals may be planned sequentially over time from the previous appointment, and should be implemented practically, according to priorities. Particular focus may be reducing intake of snack foods, which are inappropriate. The client may benefit from support of the cardiac rehabilitation team, or a local weight loss group or classes run at a local gymnasium.
- Longer-term goals include optimising an exercise regimen and achieving and maintaining an acceptable weight. If overweight, then the aim should be to reduce this by 5–10% over an acceptable time frame. The approach must continue to be reassuring.
- The client may benefit from one or two further consultations to monitor progress in dietary and lifestyle change; monitoring of cardiovascular risk parameters is appropriate (e.g. blood pressure, lipid profile).

Referral 2

- The client presents with generalised symptoms of irritable bowel syndrome, which is not unusual following an episode of gastroenteritis. Ascertaining a full picture of her dietary intake will be useful in determining any dietary intervention. A full dietary history or completed dietary records (diet diary) will guide any potential improvement in diet to assist with alleviation of symptoms. Of particular interest will be the pattern of the intake (meal and eating frequency) together with the intake of likely trigger foods/drinks (e.g. wheat-containing, milk-containing or caffeine-containing). An appreciation of the likely load of these trigger food groups will be helpful. A match of symptoms with ingestion of specific foods will be helpful (a diet diary/symptom record) and act as a baseline record to compare with any dietary changes.

- Short-term goals include improving the intake to meet healthy eating standards, and including regular amounts of macronutrients, taking frequently across the day, and checking for any change in symptoms. If the dietary pattern and intake already meet the requisites of a healthy diet, then it may be useful to target the intake towards omission of perceived food groups (this will be guided by direct questioning of the client) such as providing a dairy-free or wheat-free intake. These must be considered short-term dietary interventions, and used on a trial basis only, subject to examination of symptom records. If indeed there is connection between symptoms and intake of specific foods, then it may be worth considering a longer trial period. Any dietary intervention must be nutritionally balanced, and appropriate supplements given as necessary. It is particularly important that such radical interventions are reviewed in a timely fashion (e.g. four weekly) so that clients are not held on an overly restrictive diet without good evidence of clinical improvement.

- In the longer term, the client's progress must be reviewed: if there is no improvement in symptomatology, then the client should revert to a usual, healthy diet. If there is an improvement, then the client must be formally educated on how to manage a potentially unbalanced intake, paying specific attention to improving nutritional balance. The use of an exclusion diet to ascertain which elements of the diet may be provoking symptoms may be considered, but has a high demand on patient time and the results may not always be conclusive. Reducing stressful elements from lifestyle will assist in clinical improvement. Major dietary improvements may be achieved by alteration in eating behaviours, such as eating more slowly (eating in company) and eating more frequently (spreading intake of food across the day evenly).

Referral 3

- This client presents with overweight, which may in part be attributed to her medicine for depression (phenelzine). The client may have motivation issues stemming from depression, but she seems to be motivated ('she is keen to lose weight . . .').

- The client may be treated as any client who is overweight, but noting especially any motivating issues and respecting the prescription restrictions with use of phenelzine (avoiding foods containing tyramine, such as cheese, pickled herring, meat extracts, broad beans, yeast/soya products and game). Alcohol/low alcohol beverages must also be avoided. The drug may cause drowsiness (client should be advised to avoid driving) and dry mouth (use of sugar-free confectionery and chewing gums is helpful). Use of any herbal or complementary remedies is contraindicated. The client should be encouraged to meet usual fluid requirements (lithium).
- The diet may be planned using the basis of energy requirements and energy deficit as the principle; the diet will be based on a high intake of starchy foods and low intake of fat. The energy prescription will be based on estimation of BMR, together with a factor for PAL and the addition of an energy-deficit factor (5–700 kcal/d), resulting in a lower energy intake and one that will support reduction of weight.
- The approach taken needs to be highly motivational and must emphasise the features of healthy eating within the contexts of both modest energy restriction and restriction of foods likely to react with her medication. The client should be encouraged to engage in light physical exercise most days to assist weight control. The incidence and possible dietary causes of bloating may be investigated and dietary intervention planned around elimination of trigger foods (e.g. yeast-containing or dairy foods) and management of symptoms (such as use of pure peppermint oil/teas to buffer symptoms). The client needs to be made aware that weight loss is a slow process, and thus avoid de-motivation issues further on in the treatment, if weight loss begins to slow.
- Monitoring of weight parameters, including waist circumference and actual weight, may be useful. Compliance with dietary and lifestyle changes may be useful. The client may be offered more support than usual and reviewed in clinic on a monthly basis.

Referral 4

- Ascertaining the client's current level of knowledge and understanding about coeliac disease is an important starting point. It may be useful to explore websites visited to confirm (or otherwise) if these are peer reviewed and a reliable source of information. A diet history/diet diary prior to manipulation of diet provides valuable baseline information. A discussion about gluten in the context of wheat, barley, oats and rye (a common source of misinformation) will help to untangle some common myths.
- Modification of the diet centres on excluding sources of gluten within the context of a nutritionally balanced diet. In addition, it is useful to identify specific areas that the client may find difficult, such as managing meals out and at work and understanding how to include prescription foods as part of diet. The *Food and Drink Directory* (a check list) will be an integral part of the initial consultation.

Commentaries

- Instead of other sites on the Internet, most dietitians recommend sole use of the Coeliac UK website and information and links from this site.
- The client should be strongly recommended to join Coeliac UK (including membership with the local branch) as a major source of support (e.g. at diagnosis, the client will receive the *Food and Drink Directory*, which is an important tool in management of the disease). The client is said to be intelligent and may feel confident about interpreting food labels following the dietetic consultation, but the *Directory* will save her time and effort.
- A first review appointment may be made two weeks following initial consultation to ensure that access to prescription foods is appropriate and to offer other support. A follow-up appointment in six weeks may be useful to monitor dietary changes and discuss issues which may not have been covered because of time constraints previously, such as managing an appropriate calcium intake. A further follow-up appointment at six months may be useful to coincide with repeat endoscopy or anti-endomysial antibody determination. Local guidelines vary, but bone density should be monitored using a DEXA scanner. Further dietetic input may be necessary if there are concerns about compliance or comprehension. Monitoring should revert to annual review appointments by a health professional who is an expert in the management of coeliac disease; monitoring should include diet, BMI, urine and blood electrolytes and bone density status if appropriate (e.g. post-menopausal women). Medications, symptoms, bowel function and general well-being can also be reviewed annually.

Referral 5

- The case presents several challenges: Graves's disease (hyperthyroidism) is characterised by increased appetite and a tendency for a client to be anxious (and may affect dietary intake). The client is an overweight/obese South African gentleman, and may be used to eating large servings of meat. He appears to scavenge from food planned and prepared for his children. Attention to portion sizes and a greater emphasis on planning the client's own dietary intake may be the approach to take to reduce his energy intake. He may find increasing the amount of physical exercise rather difficult (hip complaint) to assist him with weight control.
- The client may be treated as any client who is overweight, but noting especially any motivating issues (greater mobility may relieve pain from hip complaint). Initial assessment may include a full dietary history to ascertain the positive and negative aspects of his current diet with which to plan the intervention diet.
- The diet may be planned using the basis of energy requirements and energy deficit as the principle; the diet will be based on a high intake of starchy foods and low intake of fat. The energy prescription will be based

on estimation of BMR, together with a factor for PAL and the addition of an energy-deficit factor (5–700 kcal/d), resulting in a lower energy intake and one that will support reduction of weight.

■ The approach taken needs to be motivational and must emphasise the features of healthy eating within the context of modest energy restriction. The client should be encouraged to engage in light physical exercise most days to assist weight control. The client needs to be made aware that weight loss is a slow process, and thus avoid de-motivation issues further on in the treatment, if weight loss begins to slow. Dietary intervention may wish to concentrate on portion control (especially of meat and fish) to assist with reducing energy intake. Any approach needs to take account of his emotional state and must engender confidence in self-management of the diet.

■ Monitoring of weight parameters, including waist circumference and actual weight, may be useful. Compliance with dietary and lifestyle changes may be useful. The client may be offered support to assist with weight control and reviewed every 8–10 weeks until such time as weight reduction is established.

Referral 6

■ Handling of this case may begin with a detailed dietary assessment to explore in particular the intake of NSP, fat, sugar and alcohol, and caffeine consumption. Information about meal patterns and fluid intake would also be useful. It will be important to check whether the patient has any previous experience of dietary exclusion and to note the degree of success (or otherwise). Direct questioning about the foods the patient perceives may provoke reaction, may assist in determining a way forward. Inspection of weight history/recent weight changes, together with any symptomatology (headache, fatigue) may be useful.

■ Short-term goals may include a gradual introduction of NSP (both soluble and insoluble) to recommended levels, assuming intake is poor. There is a need to increase intake of appropriate fluids, and reduce the intake of alcohol (to recommendations). Caffeine-containing foods and beverages should be omitted from the new diet. The client should be advised to increase physical activity and provided with reassurance at any outpatient appointments. There is a need to continue looking for a match between dietary intake and symptom development.

■ Longer-term goals will depend on the initial response to the above dietary changes. If there is improvement in symptoms, then reinforce the principles of a healthy eating (increased amounts of complex carbohydrate with plenty of fluids) model of dietary intake. If there is no improvement in symptoms, then a lactose-free diet may be considered. This may be implemented as a trial, and reviewed in two to four weeks. If symptoms improve then consideration of a longer-term trial (with review) may prove beneficial.

Commentaries

Referral 7

- The patient has no weight loss and has a BMI <20 kg/m² and hence shows no/little sign of nutritional depletion (loss of fat or muscle mass). However, the patient has a poor appetite and is eating less than half of his meals, and although he is not experiencing gastrointestinal symptoms, he has a high rating for stress factor. The patient is therefore at some nutritional risk. The patient will have increased nutritional requirements and will be at risk of nutritional depletion if he does not increase his dietary intake and if the illness is prolonged or if appetite is affected by any planned treatment or intervention.
- Whilst the patient may need monitoring (nursing), intervention by a dietitian may not be necessary imminently (score is a low risk). Nursing staff may need to liaise with the medical team to determine the medical treatment to be undertaken. Depending on the clinical decisions made, the patient's response, duration of treatment and length of hospital stay may all affect oral intake. It would be important for staff to evaluate clinical status, and may include monitoring temperature, clinical chemistry, albumin concentration and level of CRP. The patient does require appropriate advice about choosing items from the hospital menu that are energy-dense and high in protein.
- Appropriate approaches will include regular checking of medical/nursing notes and noting relevant clinical information/clinical chemistry. Liaison with the MDT is important to deliver consistent and informed care. Regular dietary history and/or completion of food record charts will provide important information with which to monitor voluntary oral intake. Checking the accuracy of screening information, monitoring weight history and anthropometry and looking for signs of clinical oedema are all important. The patient needs to be supported continually with choosing appropriate foods from the hospital menu, and in the provision of high energy/high protein snack foods and/or use of nutritional supplements, should appetite or weight status deteriorate.
- Nurses need to repeat the nutritional screen as protocol suggests (e.g. every three days, or weekly). The patient's weight and food intake should be monitored closely so that interventions can be adjusted according to progress.

Referral 8

- Initial assessment indicates that the patient is malnourished, with a BMI of 18 kg/m² and a weight loss of 3–6 kg. At three days post-operation oral intake still remains poor. Diarrhoea and vomiting persist and these increased fluid losses need to be replaced (fluids together with electrolytes). Post-operatively there may be a possibility of metastases and this is likely to cause a raised inflammatory response and further increase nutritional requirements. Implications of the above include: impaired recovery, impaired wound healing post-operatively, a longer hospital stay, impaired immune function (and more susceptible to hospital acquired infections) and increased risk of pressure sores.

- Management priorities will include the use of anti-emetics and pro-kinetics, short-term nasogastric feeding to improve nutritional status (meeting protein, energy and fluid requirements). Salt replacement therapy and nutritional supplements will be useful. Ultimately, use of a high energy/ high protein oral diet will be the longer-term goal; the patient may benefit from a 'little and often' eating approach.
- Monitoring will include biochemistry (urine and electrolytes) and the use of fluid balance and food record charts.

Referral 9

- The case presents as an adult male patient with no weight loss and a BMI >20 kg/m^2, who hence has no signs of nutritional depletion (i.e. fat or muscle loss). Appetite and ability to eat/retain food seem to pose no problems either. There is a moderate stress factor, which may be associated with the chronic illness or increased demands (presence of gangrene, to promote wound healing) and will increase nutritional requirements. He is at risk if he does not increase his nutritional requirements and if the illness is prolonged or his appetite/intake is affected by any planned treatment or interventions.
- Nursing staff need to liaise with the medical team to determine medical treatment to be undertaken, response to this, duration of treatment and length of hospital stay and consider how these will affect oral intake. It will be important for staff to evaluate his clinical status (temperature, clinical chemistry, albumin levels and CRP). Dietary intervention simply involves advice on selection of food from the hospital menu (high energy/ high protein, at present).
- An appropriate approach will involving noting significant documentation in the patient's medical notes and nursing notes, including clinical chemistry information. Liaison with the MDT is important. Frequent determination of intake (food record charts), assessment of the client's weight and checking accuracy of screening information is also important. Routine anthropometry, together with checking for signs of clinical oedema should be monitored. The patient should be supported to make appropriate menu choices, together with high energy/high protein snacks and use of nutritional supplements if necessary (should appetite deteriorate).
- Discharge and longer-term arrangements will include monitoring of weight, with the intention of reducing this to a realistic weight over time. He will need dietary reinforcement of an appropriate (healthy eating) diet to maintain glycaemic control. His clinical status will require review. Compliance with diet over time is also crucial.
- The client is not at a high nutritional risk unless circumstances change, and may be followed up by the community nurse or GP. It may be useful

Commentaries

to repeat nutritional screening in the community to provide some check of nutritional risk.

Referral 10

- An appropriate referral needs to be completed as per local guidelines; a referral of this nature may be because of ignorance on the part of the staff member of the guideline, or due to the pressures of time. The referral must be signed by an appropriate person and recorded on an appropriate form. This also saves the staff member time, obviating the need for searching for information or making unnecessary telephone calls. The referral must be backed up by an entry in the medical notes.
- The information required for a case such as this may include: the date of birth, diagnosis, result of tests to support diagnosis, gestational age of the baby, relevant diabetes treatment, first language of the patient, the person responsible for care, previous medical history and a brief social history.
- It is important that the patient is seen (inappropriate delay may mean that the woman commences insulin therapy prematurely or that the patient's nutritional intake is compromised). In an effort to achieve target blood glucose levels, energy intake may be reduced to sub-optimal levels, which may adversely affect growth of the baby.
- Short-term goals centre on aligning the dietary intake (with supporting lifestyle change) with clinical guidelines, and include: reducing added sugar in drinks, possible reduction in carbohydrate load at meal times, possible use of low glycaemic index foods, use of snack foods with appropriate insulin regimen and weight management appropriate for pregnancy. The nutritional intervention may centre on healthy eating with specific reference to the above points. There is also good opportunity to discuss healthy lifestyle for family and baby.
- Follow-up and monitoring arrangements will take place as part of medical ante-natal care with both diabetic and obstetric teams; usual weight and diabetic parameters will be monitored.

The commentaries: the mini-cases

Consideration of the mini-cases reveals the following observations and may help inform appropriate dietary, nutritional and lifestyle approaches and advice.

Mini-case 1

■ Clearly there is a need to assess his usual weight and the amount of weight loss over time. Assessment of whether weight loss is significant (and unintentional) is important (although the case suggests not) as this will determine the possible intervention strategy. Visual observation (subjective global assessment) may be useful, and may indicate if the patient is emaciated (although BMI is relatively high). Calculation of energy requirements will be based on BMR and may need to involve use of an appropriate stress factor (%), but this is unlikely (multiple sclerosis), and the addition of a factor for activity (however limited). Weight maintenance may be a goal; energy requirements may take account of additional energy to encourage this. Protein requirements should also be calculated using standard formulae.

■ A diet history is important and this may reveal recent dietary changes resulting in loss of weight. Assessment of swallow may be important and liaison with an SLT will be useful. Texture and modified consistency of oral diet may have to be considered. There may be a need to consider nutritional supplements to support intake. Specialised cutlery may be required to assist eating (liaison with occupational therapist). Eating should be observed to consider additional support (e.g. assistance with eating, use of ready-prepared meals). Anthropometry may be useful to monitor clinical progress, and may include MAC, ulna length and estimates of weight. Nutritional requirements should be reviewed periodically to ensure dietary goals are met (arresting weight loss and promoting target BMI).

Mini-case 2

■ There is evidence that a planned break in feeding is beneficial and will reduce the use of aspiration by allowing gastric pH to return to normal. Continuous feeding may result in the patient receiving less volume of feed over 24 hours due to interruptions and stoppages to feed. Promotion of a voluntary oral intake will reduce reliance on feeding by nasogastric means and therefore a low volume, higher energy feed delivered overnight may be indicated to encourage eating during the day. A reduction in the number of hours of feeding to allow rehabilitation and the patient to engage in greater mobility will be the benefit from freedom from tube feeding. There is a need to assess whether the patient is

Commentaries

absorbing the feed and therefore the patient needs rest from the feed to aspirate. For example, if the aspirate is less than, or equal to, 200 ml, this suggests that the patient is tolerating the feed. If higher than this, the patient may need pharmacological intervention (e.g. use of a prokinetic).

■ Discuss with the surgeon about the need to feed continuously and the case can be made (as above). It may be that the consultant does not fully appreciate the justification for implementing a rest period. If the consultant is not available, then a senior member of his team may be approached. This may be followed up with a note documented in the patient's medical notes for the medical or surgical team to clarify/follow-up. If a doctor is not available, then speaking to the senior sister who will be on the next ward round is appropriate. Any documented information should be clearly underpinned by research evidence and appropriate reference(s) cited (NICE/PENG/BAPEN).

Mini-case 3

■ Business-like approaches to weight loss may be usual in someone successful in a career; failure to lose weight and sustain weight loss may be associated with de-motivation and lack of self-esteem.

■ Refusal to be weighed may be an admission of the magnitude of problem or unwillingness to fully engage with issues of weight gain.

■ It may be important to consider a motivational approach and explore the major barriers to weight loss presented by the client.

■ A dietary assessment, or perhaps the use of a diary, may assist in influencing the nature of the therapeutic interview and formulation of subsequent dietary advice.

■ Monitoring should be considered as nutritional goals may include weight loss. Serial weight records may not be appropriate for this, or indeed any obese client, and it may be useful to consider qualitative improvements in health (e.g. looser clothes, dress size reduction, feeling better). If the client agrees it would be appropriate to measure the waist circumference.

Mini-case 4

■ Predictive equations for energy requirements in the obese subject over-estimate requirements (as based on actual weight) and their use may perpetuate obesity. It may be useful to consider calculating requirements for non-stressed individuals and adding an energy-deficit factor (400–1000 kcal/d) to encourage a decrease in energy stores or use an arbitrary judgment of 20 kcal/kg actual body weight. It may be that the MDT would have a view on management of the obese patient in critical care, but using the above, energy requirements for this patient may be based on BMR with the addition of 10–30% (bed-bound with multiple fractures) or simply by prescribing 20 kcal/kg actual bodyweight. Assuming the patient is 100 kg, and between 30 and 59 years of age, initial energy requirements may range from 2400 kcal/d (BMR = 2023 kcal + stress factor of 20% = 2023 + 405 = 2428 kcal/d) to 2000 kcal/d (using an arbitrary value to induce mobilisation of energy stores). Protein requirements may be calculated: 0.17–0.2 g(stress)/kg/d = 17–20 gN = 106–125 g protein/d. Toleration of higher intakes of protein will depend on renal/liver function. Fluid requirements are usually based on a recommendation of 35 ml/kg.

- Short-term goals centre on the patient achieving nutritional requirements and thus monitoring will be important (probably daily to begin with, and then every 48/72 hours). Since the patient is unconscious, nasogastric feeding will be required initially.
- Longer-term goals include achieving nutritional requirements but with the intention, on clinical improvement (healing and mobility), that requirements be altered to accommodate reducing body weight to achieving a normal weight BMI. The patient will eventually need to be switched from nasogastric feeding to hospital diet (with or without the use of supplementary nutrition). The patient may very well be followed up at an orthopaedic clinic; it may be wise to discharge the patient to the care of community dietitians to monitor progress with a weight reduction diet based on healthy eating and lifestyle change.

Mini-case 5

- The Internet is worldwide and may be a source of misinformation: dietary guidelines and recommendations vary between countries and foods may be named differently leading to confusion.
- A wheat-free diet is often advocated in press and websites as a treatment for food intolerances; patients may inadvertently think this is appropriate for coeliac disease (instead of a gluten-free diet).
- The patient may not have grasped that coeliac disease is a life-long condition requiring long-term management with a gluten-free diet.
- The patient may not be aware of the long-term consequences of untreated coeliac disease (e.g. osteoporosis, anaemia, malabsorption and increased risk of some forms of bowel cancer).
- The patient may not be aware of the increased requirements for dietary calcium (which may require supplementation) nor the need for regular monitoring of bone health (e.g. DEXA scanning).
- The patient may not be aware of prescribable items, especially fresh bread products (not currently available in supermarkets), which extend the range of foods available. Some other products are also not available through retail outlets.
- There is a need for regular review and monitoring.

Mini-case 6

- Compliance issues may stem from the client's age – a younger patient may not have the same appreciation of what may happen in the future (i.e. long-term complications of diabetes) and may have other priorities. Cultural background and family life are also issues. Living in a south Asian household, and not being the head of the household, Djan is unlikely to have a great deal of control over meals or indeed meal planning. The extent of dietary changes may be large (e.g. reducing amount of oil in cooking, and changing to more appropriate oils). A full understanding of the role and function of medications used as an adjunct to diet is important. Without this, an oral hypoglycaemic agent, for example, may not be taken adequately (there is evidence that Asian individuals prefer to manage without medication, unless there is a clear rationale for use). The use of Avandamet (a tablet that includes two hypoglycaemic agents – rosiglitazone and metformin) may improve clinical control. There is a potential denial of the diagnosis, and it may depend on how many family members have the condition. There is a possibility that language barriers may also exist – has the patient understood all counselling and advice clearly?

■ Clearly, ways of motivating the client to adhere to the diet need to be considered. An exploration of why the client may not be adhering to diet is required to begin the motivational approach to encourage the patient to change his dietary habits. The use of CBT techniques will help explore the client's priorities within the management of diabetes (e.g. self-monitoring methods). It is important to explore with the patient the rationale behind all aspects of his diabetes management as this may improve compliance. Involving the family in his care may assist compliance, and inviting a family member responsible for cooking and preparing food to a consultation may be useful. The help of a translator (if necessary) may assist compliance.

Mini-case 7

■ Self-referral to a dietitian may be seen as strongly motivational and a good prognosis is therefore likely.

■ Self-directed client goals (to fit a particular dress size) may strongly influence the prognosis.

■ Aggressive weight loss (10 kg in six months) may not be ethical and conflicts with evidence-based clinical guidelines.

■ The therapeutic interview should emphasise the intention to lose weight gradually and over a more realistic term in order to achieve appropriate clinical outcomes (improving health and reducing further health risk by possible inability to sustain weight loss).

Mini-case 8

■ The client presents as an underweight (BMI = 19.1 kg/m^2) elderly woman who has recently had a single hip replacement with post-operative infection.

■ It is important to check for any history of weight loss to ascertain significance of any recent unintentional weight loss. The BMI suggests evidence of nutrition depletion and this should be investigated. Short-term nutritional goals should be to ensure the patient meets nutritional requirements, especially for energy, protein and fluid. Energy should be calculated using BMR (+ stress factor for uncomplicated surgery and sepsis, say of 20%). Clearly, the patient's core temperature (WCC and CRP status) should be monitored, as sepsis with fever will increase energy requirements. Protein requirements should be calculated using prediction equations. Fluid intake is important to ensure the patient is not dehydrated (35 ml/kg).

■ In the longer term, the patient needs to be educated of the need to meet nutritional requirements, and advised of appropriate food selection (high energy/high protein) from the hospital menu, and then to planning, shopping and preparation of food at home. The patient will receive follow-up care at the orthopaedic clinic and any advice given may centre on clinical improvement or on general health information (calcium status, exercise and healthy eating). It will be appropriate to monitor weight and the extent to which the client is meeting nutritional requirements (dietary intake and compliance). Support services may be discussed in view of potential social isolation.

Mini-case 9

■ The case is rather brief, and in practice much more information is required before an adequate clinical decision can be reached. It is assumed that the client is male, probably tall (>1.82 m), with a large frame (prop forward), muscular and probably weighing about 114 kg (18 stone). These data would be ascertained prior to forming a clinical judgement. Questions that require to be known include: is the patient to be treated only for head injury? Is his gut functioning? Has the client been nil-by-mouth for the period of seven days? At what point has he been referred to the dietitian? Following confirmation of the assumed data, nutritional requirements can be calculated using predictive equations.

■ Short-term nutritional goals include providing nutritional requirements using a nasogastric tube. If he has been fed during the period of unconsciousness, then proceeding with the feed is safe. If he has not been fed, then feeding may proceed, but with adequate monitoring (re-feeding syndrome). Monitoring of urine and blood electrolytes is important and should continue until levels are stable. An appropriate feed should be selected to meet requirements. It is likely to be a high energy feed (1.5 kcal/ml). In addition, consideration of fluid requirements is important, and this will be achieved by supplying 35 ml/kg.

■ Assuming that a period of unconsciousness or prolonged rehabilitation may be necessary, consideration of a PEG feed may be justified. Prior to oral feeding, the SLT may need to assess swallow to detect any potential difficulties. Oral feeding may proceed when the client is deemed ready (with texture modification if recommended). Regular review of nutritional requirements, and the extent to which the patient is meeting these, should form the core of monitoring, including accurate weighing. Consideration of longer-term feeding may be required if the patient does not regain consciousness. Discharge planning arrangements should be discussed with medical and nursing staff, and the main aim may be home enteral feeding with home delivery of feed together with a full training package for carers and the health care professionals involved.

■ Initially monitoring should involve blood results, urine electrolytes and output and probably blood pressure (and perhaps intra-cranial pressure). Monitoring of the feed (amount delivered in relation to what is prescribed) and addressing any shortfalls will be important. Delivery of feed may be interrupted (scans, x-ray and regular physiotherapy) and relevant staff need to be kept informed.

Mini-case 10

■ Initial observations should include that the patient is an elderly man with significant and likely unintentional weight loss, which suggests the presence of malnutrition. He has been through significant episodes of surgery and treatment and likely to have been catabolic. His weight loss is associated with side-effects of treatment (affecting dietary intake and increasing nutritional requirements) including pain, fatigue, diarrhoea and/or constipation. Other medications may affect intake. If living at home he may need social support, especially if living alone.

■ Assessment suggests he is malnourished, possibly underweight and has possibly lost >10% of body weight. Additional parameters may be helpful: BMI, MUAC, TSF and these should be compared with reference ranges. Baseline data may be used to monitor nutritional status and the effects of nutritional intervention. He may be at risk of developing re-feeding syndrome.

■ Short-term nutritional goals may include ameliorating the side-effects using appropriate medications and establishing dietary advice (using a 'little and often' approach, making use of convenience foods that may be low in NSPs and ensuring adequate hydration). There is a need to prevent further unintentional weight loss. A priority will be to meet nutritional requirements (protein, energy, electrolytes, minerals, micronutrients and fluid); the use of appropriate food fortification and supplements may be indicated. Complications of nutritional support must be avoided (re-feeding syndrome) and social circumstances may be explored – he may be too tired to cook.

■ Longer-term goals may be to achieve a healthy body weight and arrest and prevent malnutrition. Healthy eating advice may reduce risk of development of future cancers and longer-standing complications managed (e.g. diarrhoea) with appropriate levels of NSPs and additional fluid. Changes in nutritional status should be recorded and additional treatment implemented as necessary.

■ Implementation of dietary intervention rests on classification of weight lost (>10% in three months) or BMI (>18.5 kg/m²) and warrants nutritional support to prevent malnutrition. Use of food fortification, oral nutritional supplements or even ANS is indicated. Actual requirements should be calculated using predictive equations; there is a need to obtain further information (age, weight, weight history and activity factor).

■ Monitoring and evaluation should begin daily, reducing to twice weekly and then three to six monthly, and may include: weight, MAC and TSF, gastrointestinal function, symptom record and any changes to the clinical condition and significant clinical chemistry. Social circumstances and compliance issues require monitoring.

The appendices: clinical information and reference data

Appendix 1 Weights and measures

Height/length

```
1 inch              = 2.54 cm
1 foot (12 inches) = 30.48 cm (0.305 m)
1 yard (36 inches) = 91.44 cm
1 centimetre       = 0.394 inch
1 metre            = 39.37 inches
```

To convert height in feet and inches to metres (e.g. a client who is 5 ft 5 inches):

(1) Convert to inches by multiplying feet by 12 and adding the additional inches:
e.g. $5 \times 12 = 60; + 5 = 65$ inches
(2) Convert to centimetres by multiplying inches by 2.54:
e.g. $65 \times 2.54 = 165.1$ cm
(3) Convert to metres by dividing by 100:
e.g. $165.1/100 = 1.651$ m

Weight/mass

```
1 ounce             = 28.35 g (in round figures, 28 g)
1 pound (16 oz)     = 454 g or 0.45 kg
1 stone (14 lb)     = 6.35 kg
1 kilogram (1000 g) = 2.2 lb
```

To convert weight in stones and pounds to kilograms (e.g. a client who is 11 st 6 lb):

(1) Convert to pounds by multiplying stones by 14 and adding the additional pounds:
e.g. $11 \times 14 = 154 + 6 = 160$ lb
(2) Convert pounds to kilograms by dividing by 2.2:
e.g. $160/2.2 = 72.7$ kg

To convert kilograms to stones and pounds (e.g. a client who is 55 kg):

(1) Multiply by 2.2:
e.g. $55 \times 2.2 = 121$ lb
(2) Divide by 14 to derive stones:
e.g. $121/14 = 8.643$ stone
(3) Multiply the fraction by 14 to derive pounds:
e.g. $0.643 \times 14 = 9.0$ lb. Imperial weight is therefore 8 stone 9 lb

Appendices

Table 1.1 Inches/centimetres conversion table.

Inches to centimetres		Centimetres to inches	
in	cm	in	cm
1	2.54	1	0.39
2	5.08	2	0.79
3	7.62	3	1.18
4	10.16	4	1.57
5	12.70	5	1.97
6	15.25	6	2.36
7	17.78	7	2.76
8	20.32	8	3.15
9	22.86	9	3.54
10	25.40	10	3.94
20	50.8	20	7.87
30	76.2	30	11.81
40	101.6	40	15.75
50	127.0	50	19.69
60	152.4	60	23.62
70	177.8	70	27.56
80	203.2	80	31.50
90	228.6	90	35.43
100	254.0	100	39.37

Volume

1 fluid ounce = 28.41 ml
1 pint (20 fl oz) = 568.3 ml (or 0.568 l)
1 litre (1000 ml) = 1.76 pints

Table 1.2 Height conversion table (feet/inches to metres).

ft	in	m	ft	in	m
4	0	1.22	5	3½	1.61
4	0½	1.23	5	4	1.63
4	1	1.24	5	4½	1.64
4	1½	1.26	5	5	1.65
4	2	1.27	5	5½	1.66
4	2½	1.28	5	6	1.68
4	3	1.29	5	6½	1.69
4	3½	1.31	5	7	1.70
4	4	1.32	5	7½	1.71
4	4½	1.33	5	8	1.73
4	5	1.35	5	8½	1.74
4	5½	1.36	5	9	1.75
4	6	1.37	5	9½	1.76
4	6½	1.38	5	10	1.78
4	7	1.40	5	10½	1.79
4	7½	1.41	5	11	1.80

Table 1.2 *Continued*

ft	in	m	ft	in	m
4	8	1.42	5	11½	1.82
4	8½	1.43	6	0	1.83
4	9	1.45	6	½	1.84
4	9½	1.46	6	1	1.85
4	10	1.47	6	1½	1.87
4	10½	1.49	6	2	1.88
4	11	1.50	6	2½	1.89
4	11½	1.51	6	3	1.90
5	0	1.52	6	3½	1.92
5	0½	1.54	6	4	1.93
5	1	1.55	6	4½	1.94
5	1½	1.56	6	5	1.96
5	2	1.57	6	5½	1.97
5	2½	1.59	6	6	1.98
5	3	1.60			

Table 1.3 Ounces/grams conversion table (approximate rounded figures).

Ounces to grams			Grams to ounces	
oz	g	(approximate conversion)	g	oz (approximate conversion)
1	28	(25–30)	10	0.35 (⅓ oz)
2	57	(50–60)	15	0.53 (½ oz)
3	85	(75–90)	20	0.71 (¾ oz)
4 (¼ lb)	113	(100–120)	30	1.06 (1 oz)
5	142	(150)	40	1.41
6	170	(175)	50	1.76 (1¾ oz)
7	198	(200)	60	2.12 (2 oz)
8 (½ lb)	227	(225)	70	2.47
9	255	(250)	80	2.82
10	284	(300)	90	3.17
11	312	(325)	100	3.53 (3½ oz)
12 (¾ lb)	340	(350)	110	3.88
13	368	(375)	120	4.23
14	397	(400)	130	4.58
15	425	(425)	140	4.94
16 (1 lb)	454	(450)	150	5.29
			175	6.31
			200	7.05
			225	7.94 (8 oz/½ lb)
			250	8.82
			300	10.58
			350	12.34 (12 oz/¾ lb)
			400	14.1
			450	15.9 (16 oz/1 lb)
			500	17.6
			1000	35.27 (2.2 lb)

Appendices

Table 1.4 Body weight conversion table (stones and pounds to kilograms).

st	lb	kg	st	lb	kg	st	lb	kg	st	lb	kg	st	lb	kg
0	1	0.45	6	5	40.37	9	13	63.05	13	7	85.73	17	1	108.41
	2	0.90		6	40.82	10	0	63.50		8	86.18		2	108.86
	3	1.36		7	41.28		1	63.96		9	86.64		3	109.32
	4	1.81		8	41.73		2	64.41		10	87.09		4	109.77
	5	2.27		9	42.18		3	64.86		11	87.54		5	110.22
	6	2.72		10	42.64		4	65.32		12	88.00		6	110.68
	7	3.17		11	43.09		5	65.77		13	88.45		7	111.13
	8	3.63		12	43.55		6	66.23	14	0	88.91		8	111.59
	9	4.08		13	44.00		7	66.68		1	89.36		9	112.04
	10	4.54	7	0	44.45		8	67.13		2	89.81		10	112.49
	11	4.99		1	44.91		9	67.59		3	90.27		11	112.95
	12	5.44		2	45.36		10	68.04		4	90.72		12	113.40
	13	5.90		3	45.81		11	68.49		5	91.17		13	113.85
				4	46.27		12	68.95		6	91.63	18	0	114.31
1	0	6.35		5	46.72		13	69.40		7	92.08		1	114.76
2	0	12.70		6	47.17	11	0	69.85		8	92.53		2	115.21
3	0	19.05		7	47.63		1	70.31		9	92.98		3	115.67
4	0	25.40		8	48.08		2	70.76		10	93.44		4	116.12
	1	25.86		9	48.54		3	71.22		11	93.90		5	116.58
	2	26.31		10	48.99		4	71.67		12	94.35		6	117.03
	3	26.76		11	49.44		5	72.12		13	94.80		7	117.48
	4	27.22		12	49.90		6	72.58	15	0	95.26		8	117.94
	5	27.67		13	50.35		7	73.03		1	95.71		9	118.39
	6	28.12	8	0	50.80		8	73.48		2	96.16		10	118.84
	7	28.57		1	51.26		9	73.94		3	96.62		11	119.30
	8	29.03		2	51.71		10	74.39		4	97.07		12	119.75
	9	29.48		3	52.16		11	74.84		5	97.52		13	120.20
	10	29.93		4	52.62		12	75.30		6	97.98	19	0	120.66
	11	30.39		5	53.07		13	75.75		7	98.43		1	121.11
	12	30.84		6	53.52	12	0	76.20		8	98.88		2	121.56
	13	31.30		7	53.98		1	76.66		9	99.34		3	122.02
5	0	31.75		8	54.43		2	77.11		10	99.79		4	122.47
	1	32.21		9	54.89		3	77.57		11	100.24		5	122.93
	2	32.66		10	55.34		4	78.02		12	100.70		6	123.38
	3	33.11		11	55.79		5	78.47		13	101.15		7	123.83
	4	33.57		12	56.25		6	78.93	16	0	101.61		8	124.29
	5	34.02		13	56.70		7	79.38		1	102.06		9	124.74
	6	34.47	9	0	57.15		8	79.83		2	102.51		10	125.19
	7	34.93		1	57.61		9	80.29		3	102.97		11	125.65
	8	35.38		2	58.06		10	80.74		4	103.42		12	126.10
	9	35.83		3	58.51		11	81.19		5	103.87		13	126.55
	10	36.29		4	58.97		12	81.65		6	104.33	20	0	127.27
	11	36.74		5	59.42		13	82.10		7	104.79		7	130.45
	12	37.19		6	59.88	13	0	82.55		8	105.24	21	0	133.64
	13	37.65		7	60.33		1	83.01		9	105.69		7	136.82
6	0	38.10		8	60.78		2	83.46		10	106.14	22	0	140.00
	1	38.56		9	61.24		3	83.92		11	106.60		7	143.18
	2	39.01		10	61.69		4	84.37		12	107.04	23	0	146.36
	3	39.46		11	62.14		5	84.82		13	107.50	24	0	152.73
	4	39.92		12	62.60		6	85.28	17	0	107.96	25	0	159.09

Table 1.5 Pints/litres conversion table.

fl oz/pints	ml/litres	(approximate measure)	ml/litres	fl oz/pints
1 fl oz	28	(25)	50 ml	1.75 fl oz
¼ pint (5 fl oz)	142	(150)	100 ml	3.5 fl oz
½ pint (10 fl oz)	284	(275)	200 ml	7 fl oz
¾ pint (15 fl oz)	426	(425)	250 ml	8.8 fl oz
1 pint	568	(550)	500 ml	17.6 fl oz
2 pints	1.1 litres		750 ml	26.4 fl oz
3 pints	1.7 litres		1 litre	1.76 pints (1¾ pints)
4 pints	2.3 litres			
5 pints	2.8 litres			

Appendix 2 Dietary data

Conversion factors

(1)   Energy

Conversion factors for kilocalories to kilojoules/megajoules

1 kilocalorie (kcal)   = 4.184 kilojoules (kJ)
1000 kcal   = 4.184 megajoules (MJ)
1 kilojoule   = 0.239 kcal
1 megajoule (1000 kJ) = 239 kcal

For converting the energy content of diets of normal composition, a conversion factor of 1 kcal = 4.2 kJ can be used

To convert:

kcal to kJ	Multiply by 4.2
kcal to MJ	Multiply by 4.2/1000
	or
	Divide by 239
kJ to kcal	Divide by 4.2
MJ to kcal	Divide by 4.2/1000
	or
	Multiply by 239

(2)   Protein/nitrogen

Protein g   = nitrogen g × 6.25*
Nitrogen g = protein g/6.25*

* This conversion factor is only appropriate for a mixture of foods. For milk or cereals alone, the factor 6.4 or 5.7, respectively, should be used.

Nitrogen balance

Nitrogen input g = protein g taken in 24 hours/6.25
Nitrogen output g = nitrogen g lost in urine + 2–4 g (obligatory nitrogen
                    losses in skin and faeces)
Nitrogen balance = nitrogen input – nitrogen output

Table 2.1 Energy yields from nutrients.

Nutrient	Energy yield per gram	
	kcal	kJ
Protein	4	17
Fat	9	37
Carbohydrate	3.75	16
Alcohol	7	29
Medium-chain triglyceride (MCT)	8.4	35

(3) Vitamin A

The active vitamin A content of the diet is usually expressed in retinol equivalents:

1 µg retinol equivalent = 1 µg retinol or 6 µg β-carotene equivalents
µg retinol equivalents = µg retinol + (µg β-carotene equivalents/6)

Occasionally the vitamin A content of foods is still expressed in international units (i.u.):
1 i.u = 0.3 µg retinol (or 0.6 µg carotene equivalents)

(4) Vitamin D

1 µg vitamin D = 40 international units (i.u.)
1 i.u.   = 0.025 µg vitamin D

To convert:

µg vitamin D to i.u.   Multiply by 40
i.u. vitamin D to µg   Divide by 40

(5) Vitamin E

Vitamin E activity is expressed as D-α-tocopherol equivalents. Where activity is given in international units (i.u.): 1 i.u. is equivalent to 0.67 mg D-α-tocopherol.

(6) Nicotinic acid/tryptophan

1 mg nicotinic acid can be produced from 60 mg tryptophan.
Nicotinic acid mg equivalents = nicotinic acid mg + (tryptophan mg/60)

Food exchange lists

(1) Carbohydrate

Table 2.2 Food portions containing approximately 10g carbohydrate.

Food	Portion providing about 10g carbohydrate	Approximate energy content (kcal)
White bread	20g (one large thin slice)	50
Wholemeal bread	25g (one small thin slice)	50
Wholewheat breakfast cereal	20g (5 tablespoons)	50
Cornflakes/plain breakfast cereal	10g (5 tablespoons)	40
Muesli	15g (2 tablespoons)	50
Rice (cooked)	30g (one tablespoon)	40
Pasta (cooked)	50g (2 tablespoons)	50
Baked beans	70g (3 tablespoons)	60
Potato (boiled)	50g (one egg-sized)	40
Potato (chips)	25g (4 large chips)	65
Milk	200ml	130 (full-fat) 90 (semi-skimmed) 65 (skimmed)
Fresh fruit	120–150g (one medium-sized piece of fruit or serving)	50
Dried fruit	15g (one tablespoon)	40
Unsweetened fruit juice	100ml (one wine-glass)	40
Digestive biscuits	15g (one biscuit)	70
Plain/semi-sweet biscuits	15g (2 biscuits)	60
Sponge cake	20g	90
Fruit cake	16g	60
Sugar-containing soft drink (squash/fizzy)	100ml (small glass)	40
Pastry	15g	80
Flour	10g	40

(2) Protein

Table 2.3 Food portions containing approximately 6 or 2g protein.

Food	Portion size	Protein/ portion (g)	Approximate energy/ portion (kcal)
Milk	180ml	6	115 (full-fat) 85 (semi-skimmed) 60 (skimmed)
Cheddar cheese	25g	6	100
Yogurt	125g	6	125
Egg	50g (one small egg)	6	70
Meat/poultry lean cooked	25g	6	40
White fish	35g	6	30
Baked beans	120g	6	100
Peas	100g	6	70
Bread (1 large thin slice)	25g	2	50
Pasta (boiled)	50g	2	50
Rice (boiled)	100g	2	140
Most breakfast cereals	25g	2	90
Digestive biscuits	15g (one biscuit)	2	70
Potatoes	140g	2	100
Crisps	30g	2	160

(3) Potassium

Table 2.4 Food portions containing approximately 4 mmol potassium.

Food	Portion size providing approximately 4 mmol potassium	Food	Portion size providing approximately 4 mmol potassium
Milk	100 ml	Wholemeal bread	70 g
Yogurt	60 g	Apple	125 g
Cheddar cheese	130 g	Orange with skin	100 g
Egg	100 g (2 small eggs)	Grapes/orange without skin	50 g
Meat/fish	50 g	Potato boiled	50 g
White flour	120 g	Orange juice	100 ml
Wholemeal flour	45 g	Tomato juice	60 ml
White bread	160 g		

(4) Sodium

Table 2.5 Sodium/salt-restricted diets.

No added salt
This restricts sodium intake to less than 100 mmol Na⁺/day
A pinch of salt may be used in cooking, but none should be added to food at the table
The following foods must be avoided:

- Bacon, ham, sausages, paté
- Tinned fish and meat
- Smoked fish and meat
- Fish and meat pastes
- Tinned and packet soups
- Sauce mixes
- Tinned vegetables
- Bottled sauces and chutneys
- Meat and vegetable extracts, stock cubes
- Salted nuts and crisps
- Soya sauce
- Monosodium glutamate
- Cheese – up to 100 g per week
- Bread – up to 4 slices per day

40 mmol Sodium diet
In addition to the 'No added salt' foods listed, the following restrictions apply:

- No salt to be used in cooking or at table
- Salt-free butter or margarine must be used
- Milk should be restricted to 300 ml per day
- Breakfast cereals must be salt-free

E number classification system

E100–180	Colours	E322–495	Emulsifiers/stabilisers/acidity regulators/thickeners
E200–283	Preservatives		
E300–321	Antioxidants	E950–969	Artificial sweeteners

Table 2.6 Commonly used additives.

Type of additive	E number	Chemical name
Colours	E101	Riboflavin (yellow)
Natural/nature identical colours	E100	Curcumin (yellow)
	E120	Cochineal (red)
	E140	Chlorophyll (green)
	E150a	Plain caramel (brown/black)
	E153	Carbon (black)
	E160a	α-, β- and γ-carotene (yellow/orange)
	E160b	Annatto (yellow/red)
	E160c	Capsanthin (paprika extract) (red/orange)
	E160d	Lycopene (red extract from tomatoes)
	E162	Beetroot red (betanin) (purple/red)
	E163	Anthocyanins (red/blue/violet)
Synthetic colours	E102	Tartrazine* (yellow)
	E104	Quinoline Yellow*
	E110	Sunset Yellow FCF*
	E122	Carmoisine (azorubine) * (red)
	E123	Amaranth* (purple red)
	E124	Ponceau 4R* (red)
	E127	Erythrosine* (pink/red)
	E128	Red 2G*
	E129	Allura Red AC*
	E132	Indigo carmine (indigotine)* (blue)
	E142	Green S*
	E150b–d	Caustic sulphite caramel; ammonia caramel; sulphite ammonia caramel (brown/black)
	E151	Black PN*
	E154	Brown FK*
	E155	Brown HT*
	E180	Litholrubine BK (pigment rubine; rubine)*
Preservatives	E200	Sorbic acid
Sorbic acid and its derivatives	E201–E203	Sodium, potassium and calcium sorbates
Benzoic acid and derivatives	E210	Benzoic acid
	E211–E213	Sodium, potassium and calcium benzoates
	E214–E219	Ethyl, methyl and propyl hydroxybenzoates
Sulphur dioxide and derivatives	E220	Sulphur dioxide
	E221	Sodium sulfite
	E222	Sodium hydrogensulfite (sodium bisulfite)

Table 2.6 *Continued*

Type of additive	E number	Chemical name
	E223	Sodium metabisulfite
	E224	Potassium metabisulfite
	E226	Calcium sulfite
	E227	Calcium hydrogensulfite (calcium bisulfite)
Nitrites and nitrates	E249	Potassium nitrite
	E250	Sodium nitrite
	E251	Sodium nitrate
	E252	Potassium nitrate
Acetic, lactic and propionic acid derivatives	E260–E263	Acetic acid and acetates
	E270	Lactic acid
	E280–E283	Propionic acid and propionates
Antioxidants		
Ascorbic acid and derivatives	E300	Ascorbic acid (vitamin C)
	E301–E304	Ascorbates and ascorbyl palmitate
Tocopherols	E306	Vitamin E
	E307–E309	Synthetic tocopherols
Gallates	E310–E312	Propyl, octyl and dodecyl gallates
BHA /BHT	E320	Butylated hydroxyanisole (BHA)
	E321	Butylated hydroxytoluene (BHT)
Emulsifiers and stabilisers		
Emulsifier	E322	Lecithins
Acidity regulators, buffers, stabilisers	E325–E327	Sodium, potassium and calcium lactate
	E330–E333	Citric acid; sodium, potassium and calcium citrates
	E334–E337	Tartaric acid; sodium and potassium tartrates
	E338–E341	Phosphoric acid; sodium, potassium and calcium phosphates and orthophosphates
	E350–E352	Sodium, potassium and calcium malates
Gelling agents	E401–E405	Sodium, ammonium, potassium and calcium alginates
	E406	Agar
	E407	Carrageenan
Gums	E410	Locust bean gum
	E412	Guar gum
	E413	Tragacanth
	E414	Gum arabic
	E415	Xanthan gum
Emulsifiers/stabilisers	E471–E477	Esters and glycerides of fatty acids (e.g. mono- and diglycerides of fatty acids or glyceryl monostearate and distearate)

*Azo dye.

Appendix 3 Body mass index

$$\text{Body mass index (BMI)} = \frac{\text{weight in kg}}{(\text{height in m})^2}$$

Interpretation of BMI:

<16	Severely underweight
16–19	Underweight
20–25	Normal range
26–30	Overweight
31–40	Obese
>40	Morbidly obese

An accompanying waist circumference >94 cm (37 inches) in men and >80 cm (32 inches) in women is indicative of central obesity.

Appendices

Table 3.1 BMI ready reference table.

	BMI	Weight (kg)																						
Morbidly obese (BMI > 40)	45	102	104	107	110	113	116	119	121	124	127	131	134	137	140	143	146	150	153	156	159	163	170	173
	44	99	102	105	108	110	113	116	119	122	125	128	131	134	137	140	143	146	149	153	156	159	166	169
	43	97	100	102	105	108	111	113	116	119	122	125	128	131	134	137	140	143	146	149	152	156	162	166
	42	95	97	100	103	105	108	111	113	116	119	122	125	128	131	134	137	140	143	146	149	152	159	162
	41	93	95	98	100	103	105	108	111	113	116	119	122	125	127	130	133	136	139	142	145	148	155	158
Obese (BMI 31–40)	40	90	93	95	98	100	103	105	108	111	113	116	119	122	124	127	130	133	136	139	142	145	151	154
	39	88	91	93	95	98	100	103	105	108	111	113	116	119	121	124	127	130	132	135	138	141	147	150
	38	86	88	91	93	95	98	100	103	105	108	110	113	115	118	121	124	126	129	132	135	138	143	146
	37	84	86	88	90	93	95	98	100	102	105	107	110	112	115	118	120	123	126	128	131	134	140	143
	36	81	84	86	88	90	93	95	97	100	102	104	107	109	112	115	117	120	122	125	128	130	136	139
	35	79	81	83	86	88	90	92	95	97	99	102	104	106	109	111	114	116	119	122	124	127	132	135
	34	77	79	81	83	85	87	90	92	94	96	99	101	103	106	108	111	113	116	118	121	123	128	131
	33	75	77	79	81	83	85	87	89	91	94	96	98	100	103	105	107	110	112	115	117	120	125	127
	32	72	74	76	78	80	82	84	87	89	91	93	95	97	100	102	104	106	109	111	114	116	121	123
	31	70	72	74	76	78	80	82	84	86	88	90	92	94	96	99	101	103	105	108	110	112	117	120
Overweight (BMI 26–30)	30	68	70	72	73	75	77	79	81	83	85	87	89	91	93	96	98	100	102	104	106	109	113	116
	29	66	67	69	71	73	75	77	78	80	82	84	86	88	90	92	94	97	99	101	103	105	110	112
	28	63	65	67	69	70	72	74	76	78	79	81	83	85	87	89	91	93	95	97	99	102	106	108
	27	61	63	64	66	68	70	71	73	75	77	78	80	82	84	86	88	90	92	94	96	98	102	104
	26	59	61	62	64	65	67	69	70	72	74	76	77	79	81	83	85	87	88	90	92	94	98	100
Normal weight (BMI 20–25)	25	57	58	60	61	63	64	66	68	69	71	73	74	76	78	80	81	83	85	87	89	91	95	96
	24	54	56	57	59	60	62	63	65	67	68	70	71	73	75	76	78	80	82	83	85	87	91	93
	23	52	54	55	56	58	59	61	62	64	65	67	68	70	72	73	75	77	78	80	82	83	87	89
	22	50	51	53	54	55	57	58	60	61	63	64	66	67	69	70	72	73	75	77	78	80	83	85
	21	48	49	50	52	53	54	56	57	58	60	61	63	64	65	67	68	70	72	73	75	76	79	81
	20	45	47	48	49	50	52	53	54	56	57	58	60	61	62	64	65	67	68	70	71	73	76	77
Underweight (BMI 16–19)	19	43	44	46	47	48	49	50	52	53	54	55	57	58	59	61	62	63	65	66	68	69	72	73
	18	41	42	43	44	45	47	48	49	50	51	52	54	55	56	57	59	60	61	63	64	65	68	70
	17	39	40	41	42	43	44	45	46	47	48	50	51	52	53	54	56	57	58	59	61	62	64	66
	16	36	37	38	39	40	41	42	43	45	46	47	48	49	50	51	52	53	55	56	57	58	61	62
Severely underweight (BMI < 16)	15	34	35	36	37	38	39	40	41	42	43	44	45	46	47	48	49	50	51	52	53	55	57	58
	14	32	33	34	35	35	36	37	38	39	40	41	42	43	44	45	46	47	48	49	50	51	53	54
	13	30	30	31	32	33	34	35	35	36	37	38	39	40	41	42	43	44	44	45	46	47	49	50
	12	27	28	29	30	30	31	32	33	34	34	35	36	37	38	38	39	40	41	42	43	44	46	47
	11	25	26	27	27	28	29	29	30	31	31	32	33	34	35	35	36	37	38	39	39	40	42	43
	10	23	24	24	25	25	26	27	27	28	29	29	30	31	31	32	33	34	34	35	36	37	38	39
Height (m)		1.5	1.52	1.54	1.56	1.58	1.6	1.62	1.64	1.66	1.68	1.7	1.72	1.74	1.76	1.78	1.8	1.82	1.84	1.86	1.88	1.9	1.94	1.96
Height (feet inches)		4 11	5 0	5 1	5 1½	5 2¼	5 3	5 3¼	5 4½	5 5½	5 6	5 7	5 7¼	5 8½	5 9¼	5 10	5 11	5 11¾	60½	61¼	6 2	6 3	6 4½	6 5½

Appendix 4 Anthropometric data

Demiquet and mindex

These can be used as an index of adiposity in elderly people.

$$\text{Demiquest} = \frac{\text{weight in kg}}{(\text{demispan in m})^2}$$

$$\text{Mindex} = \frac{\text{weight in kg}}{\text{demispan in m}}$$

Table 4.1 Distribution of Demiquet and Mindex in a normal population over the age of 65 years. Data derived from Lehmann *et al.* (1991).

	Percentile				
	10th	30th	50th	70th	90th
Men (Demiquet kg/m²)					
64–74 years	87.6	99.6	106.7	117.1	130.7
75+ years	84.5	98.9	106.3	113.4	125.0
Women (Mindex kg/m)					
64–74 years	68.3	77.8	84.8	92.3	110.6
75+ years	63.1	73.6	81.7	88.4	102.2

Upper arm anthropometry

For measurement techniques and discussion.

Table 4.2 Triceps skinfold thickness (TSF). Data derived from Bishop *et al.* (1981).

Age (years)	Mean (mm)	Centile						
		5th	10th	25th	50th	75th	90th	95th
Men								
18–74	**12.0**	**4.5**	**6.0**	**8.0**	**11.0**	**15.0**	**20.0**	**23.0**
18–24	11.2	4.0	5.0	7.0	9.5	14.0	20.0	23.0
25–34	12.6	4.5	5.5	8.0	12.0	16.0	21.5	24.0
35–44	12.4	5.0	6.0	8.5	12.0	15.5	20.0	23.0
45–54	12.4	5.0	6.0	8.0	11.0	15.0	20.0	25.5
55–64	11.6	5.0	6.0	8.0	11.0	14.0	18.0	21.5
65–74	11.8	4.5	5.5	8.0	11.0	15.0	19.0	22.0
Women								
18–74	**23.0**	**11.0**	**13.0**	**17.0**	**22.0**	**28.0**	**34.0**	**37.5**
18–24	19.4	9.4	11.0	14.0	18.0	24.0	30.0	34.0
25–34	21.9	10.5	12.0	16.0	21.0	26.5	33.5	37.0
35–44	24.0	12.0	14.0	18.0	23.0	29.5	35.5	39.0
45–54	25.4	13.0	15.0	20.0	25.0	30.0	36.0	40.0
55–64	24.9	11.0	14.0	19.0	25.0	30.5	35.0	39.0
65–74	23.3	11.5	14.0	18.0	23.0	28.0	33.0	36.0

Appendices

Table 4.3 Mid-arm circumference (MAC). Data derived from Bishop *et al.* (1981).

Age (years)	Mean (mm)	Centile						
		5th	10th	25th	50th	75th	90th	95th
Men								
18–74	**31.8**	**26.4**	**27.6**	**29.6**	**31.7**	**33.9**	**36.0**	**37.3**
18–24	30.9	25.7	27.1	28.7	30.7	32.9	35.5	37.4
25–34	30.5	25.3	26.5	28.5	30.7	32.4	34.4	35.5
35–44	32.3	27.0	28.2	30.0	32.0	34.4	36.5	37.6
45–54	32.7	27.8	28.7	30.7	32.7	34.8	36.3	37.1
55–64	32.1	26.7	27.8	30.0	32.0	34.2	36.2	37.6
65–74	31.5	25.6	27.3	29.6	31.7	33.4	35.2	36.6
Women								
18–74	**29.4**	**23.2**	**24.3**	**26.2**	**28.7**	**31.9**	**35.2**	**37.8**
18–24	27.0	22.1	23.0	24.5	26.4	28.8	31.7	34.3
25–34	28.6	23.3	24.2	25.7	27.8	30.4	34.1	37.2
35–44	30.0	24.1	25.2	26.8	29.2	32.2	36.2	38.5
45–54	30.7	24.3	25.7	27.5	30.3	32.9	36.8	39.3
55–64	30.7	23.9	25.1	27.7	30.2	33.3	36.3	38.2
65–74	30.1	23.8	25.2	27.4	29.9	32.5	35.3	37.2

Table 4.4 Mid-arm muscle circumference (MAMC). Data derived from Bishop *et al.* (1981).
MAMC (cm) = MAC (cm) − [TSF (mm) × 0.314]

Age (years)	Mean (mm)	Centile						
		5th	10th	25th	50th	75th	90th	95th
Men								
18–74	**28.0**	**23.8**	**24.8**	**26.3**	**27.9**	**29.6**	**31.4**	**32.5**
18–24	27.4	23.5	24.4	25.8	27.2	28.9	30.8	32.3
25–34	28.3	24.2	25.3	26.5	28.0	30.0	31.7	32.9
35–44	28.8	25.0	25.6	27.1	28.7	30.3	32.1	33.0
45–54	28.2	24.0	24.9	26.5	28.1	29.8	31.5	32.6
55–64	27.8	22.8	24.4	26.2	27.9	29.6	31.0	31.8
65–74	26.8	22.5	23.7	25.3	26.9	28.5	29.9	30.7
Women								
18–74	**22.2**	**18.4**	**19.0**	**20.2**	**21.8**	**23.6**	**25.8**	**27.4**
18–24	20.9	17.7	18.5	19.4	20.6	22.1	23.6	24.9
25–34	21.7	18.3	18.9	20.0	21.4	22.9	24.9	26.6
35–44	22.5	18.5	19.2	20.6	22.0	24.0	26.1	27.4
45–54	22.7	18.8	19.5	20.7	22.2	24.3	26.6	27.8
55–64	22.8	18.6	19.5	20.8	22.6	24.4	26.3	28.1
65–74	22.8	18.6	19.5	20.8	22.5	24.4	26.5	28.1

Table 4.5 Dynamometry (grip strength). Data derived from Klidjian *et al.* (1980) and Griffith and Clark (1984).

Age (years)	Normal values (kg)	85% of normal (kg) (values at or below this level are indicative of protein malnutrition)
Men		
18–69	40.0	34.0
70–79	32.5	27.5
80+	22.5	19.0
Women		
18–69	27.5	23.0
70–79	25.0	21.0
80+	20.0	17.0

Estimating height from ulna length

Table 4.6 Estimates of height from ulna length, Elia (2003).

Men: height (m)		Ulna length (cm)	Women: height (m)	
<65 years	>65 years		<65 years	>65 years
1.94	1.87	32.0	1.84	1.84
1.93	1.86	31.5	1.83	1.83
1.91	1.84	31.0	1.81	1.81
1.89	1.82	30.5	1.80	1.79
1.87	1.81	30.0	1.79	1.78
1.85	1.79	29.5	1.77	1.76
1.84	1.78	29.0	1.76	1.75
1.82	1.76	28.5	1.75	1.73
1.80	1.75	28.0	1.73	1.71
1.78	1.73	27.5	1.72	1.70
1.76	1.71	27.0	1.70	1.68
1.75	1.70	26.5	1.69	1.66
1.73	1.68	26.0	1.68	1.65
1.71	1.67	25.5	1.66	1.63
1.69	1.65	25.0	1.65	1.61
1.67	1.63	24.5	1.63	1.60
1.66	1.62	24.0	1.62	1.58
1.64	1.60	23.5	1.61	1.56
1.62	1.59	23.0	1.59	1.55
1.60	1.57	22.5	1.58	1.53
1.58	1.56	22.0	1.56	1.52
1.57	1.54	21.5	1.55	1.50
1.55	1.52	21.0	1.54	1.48
1.53	1.51	20.5	1.52	1.47
1.51	1.49	20.0	1.51	1.45
1.49	1.48	19.5	1.50	1.44
1.48	1.46	19.0	1.48	1.42
1.46	1.45	18.5	1.47	1.40

Appendices

References

Bishop CW, Bowen PE, Ritchey SJ. Norms for nutritional assessment of American adults by upper arm anthropometry. *American Journal of Clinical Nutrition* 1981; **34**: 2530–2539.

Elia M. *Development and Use of the Malnutrition Universal Screening Tool ('MUST') for adults.* Redditch: BAPEN, 2003.

Griffith CD, Clark RD. A comparison of the 'Sheffield' Prognostic Index with forearm muscle dynamometry in patients from Sheffield undergoing major abdominal and urological surgery. *Clinical Nutrition* 1984; **3**: 147–151.

Klidjian AM, Foster KJ, Kammerling RM, Cooper A, Karran SJ. Relation of anthropometric and dynamometric variables to serious postoperative complications. *British Medical Journal* 1980; **281**: 899–901.

Lehmann AB, Bassey EJ, Morgan K, Dallosso HM. Normal values for weight, skeletal size and body mass indices in 890 men and women aged over 65 years. *Clinical Nutrition* 1991; **10**: 18–22.

Appendix 5 Predicting energy requirements

In the clinical setting, an estimate of an individual's energy requirements can be obtained by:

(1) Estimating the basal metabolic rate (BMR).
(2) Adding appropriate factors for stress.
(3) Adding a combined factor for activity and diet-induced thermogenesis.

The resulting estimate may need to be adjusted in order to increase or decrease body weight.

Basal metabolic rate

Basal metabolic rate (BMR) can be calculated by means of the equations summarised in Table 5.1. Alternatively, the BMR ready reckoner in Table 5.2 can be used.

Table 5.1 Schofield prediction equations for estimation of BMR. Based on DH (1991).

| Age range (years) | BMR (kcal/24 hours) | |
	Males	Females
10–17	(17.7 × kg body wt) + 657	(13.4 × kg body wt) + 692
18–29	(15.1 × kg body wt) + 692	(14.8 × kg body wt) + 487
30–59	(11.5 × kg body wt) + 873	(8.3 × kg body wt) + 846
60–74	(11.9 × kg body wt) + 700	(9.2 × kg body wt) + 687
75+	(8.4 × kg body wt) + 821	(9.8 × kg body wt) + 624

Table 5.2 Basal metabolic rate (BMR) ready reckoner. This table enables the BMR (kcal/24 hours) of a healthy individual to be predicted from weight and age.

Weight (kg)	Men (age, years)					Women (age, years)				
	10–17	18–29	30–59	60–74	74+	10–17	18–29	30–59	60–74	74+
25	1100	1070	1161	998	1031	1027	857	1054	917	869
26	1117	1085	1172	1009	1039	1040	872	1062	926	879
27	1135	1100	1184	1021	1048	1054	887	1070	935	889
28	1153	1115	1195	1033	1056	1067	901	1078	945	898
29	1170	1130	1207	1045	1065	1081	916	1087	954	908
30	1188	1145	1218	1057	1073	1094	931	1095	963	918
31	1206	1160	1230	1069	1081	1107	946	1103	972	928
32	1223	1175	1241	1081	1090	1121	961	1112	981	938
33	1241	1190	1253	1093	1098	1134	975	1120	991	947
34	1259	1205	1264	1105	1107	1148	990	1128	1000	957
35	1277	1221	1276	1117	1115	1161	1005	1137	1009	967
36	1294	1236	1287	1128	1123	1174	1020	1145	1018	977
37	1312	1251	1299	1140	1132	1188	1035	1153	1027	987
38	1330	1266	1310	1152	1140	1201	1049	1161	1037	996
39	1347	1281	1322	1164	1149	1215	1064	1170	1046	1006
40	1365	1296	1333	1176	1157	1228	1079	1178	1055	1016
41	1383	1311	1345	1188	1165	1241	1094	1186	1064	1026
42	1400	1326	1356	1200	1174	1255	1109	1195	1073	1036
43	1418	1341	1368	1212	1182	1268	1123	1203	1083	1045
44	1436	1356	1379	1224	1191	1282	1138	1211	1092	1055
45	1454	1372	1391	1236	1199	1295	1153	1220	1101	1065
46	1471	1387	1402	1247	1207	1308	1168	1228	1110	1075
47	1489	1402	1414	1259	1216	1322	1183	1236	1119	1085
48	1507	1417	1425	1271	1224	1335	1197	1244	1129	1094
49	1524	1432	1437	1283	1233	1349	1212	1253	1138	1104
50	1542	1447	1448	1295	1241	1362	1227	1261	1147	1114
51	1560	1462	1460	1307	1249	1375	1242	1269	1156	1124
52	1577	1477	1471	1319	1258	1389	1257	1278	1165	1134
53	1595	1492	1483	1331	1266	1402	1271	1286	1175	1143
54	1613	1507	1494	1343	1275	1416	1286	1294	1184	1153
55	1631	1523	1506	1355	1283	1429	1301	1303	1193	1163
56	1648	1538	1517	1366	1291	1442	1316	1311	1202	1173
57	1666	1553	1529	1378	1300	1456	1331	1319	1211	1183
58	1684	1568	1540	1390	1308	1469	1345	1327	1221	1192
59	1701	1583	1552	1402	1317	1483	1360	1336	1230	1202
60	1719	1598	1563	1414	1325	1496	1375	1344	1239	1212
61	1737	1613	1575	1426	1333	1509	1390	1352	1248	1222
62	1754	1628	1586	1438	1342	1523	1405	1361	1257	1232
63	1772	1643	1598	1450	1350	1536	1419	1369	1267	1241
64	1790	1658	1609	1462	1359	1550	1434	1377	1276	1251
65	1808	1674	1621	1474	1367	1563	1449	1386	1285	1261
66	1825	1689	1632	1485	1375	1576	1464	1394	1294	1271
67	1843	1704	1644	1497	1384	1590	1479	1402	1303	1281
68	1861	1719	1655	1509	1392	1603	1493	1410	1313	1290
69	1878	1734	1667	1521	1401	1617	1508	1419	1322	1300
70	1896	1749	1678	1533	1409	1630	1523	1427	1331	1310
71	1914	1764	1690	1545	1417	1643	1538	1435	1340	1320
72	1931	1779	1701	1557	1426	1657	1553	1444	1349	1330
73	1949	1794	1713	1569	1434	1670	1567	1452	1359	1339
74	1967	1809	1724	1581	1443	1684	1582	1460	1368	1349
75	1985	1825	1736	1593	1451	1697	1597	1469	1377	1359
76	2002	1840	1747	1604	1459	1710	1612	1477	1386	1369

Table 5.2 *Continued*

Weight (kg)	Men (age, years)					Women (age, years)				
	10–17	18–29	30–59	60–74	74+	10–17	18–29	30–59	60–74	74+
77	2020	1855	1759	1616	1468	1724	1627	1485	1395	1379
78	2038	1870	1770	1628	1476	1737	1641	1493	1405	1388
79	2055	1885	1782	1640	1485	1751	1656	1502	1414	1398
80	2073	1900	1793	1652	1493	1764	1671	1510	1423	1408
81	2091	1915	1805	1664	1501	1777	1686	1518	1432	1418
82	2108	1930	1816	1676	1510	1791	1701	1527	1441	1428
83	2126	1945	1828	1688	1518	1804	1715	1535	1451	1437
84	2144	1960	1839	1700	1527	1818	1730	1543	1460	1447
85	2162	1976	1851	1712	1535	1831	1745	1552	1469	1457
86	2179	1991	1862	1723	1543	1844	1760	1560	1478	1467
87	2197	2006	1874	1735	1552	1858	1775	1568	1487	1477
88	2215	2021	1885	1747	1560	1871	1789	1576	1497	1486
89	2232	2036	1897	1759	1569	1885	1804	1585	1506	1496
90	2250	2051	1908	1771	1577	1898	1819	1593	1515	1506
91	2268	2066	1920	1783	1585	1911	1834	1601	1524	1516
92	2285	2081	1931	1795	1594	1925	1849	1610	1533	1526
93	2303	2096	1943	1807	1602	1938	1863	1618	1543	1535
94	2321	2111	1954	1819	1611	1952	1878	1626	1552	1545
95	2339	2127	1966	1831	1619	1965	1893	1635	1561	1555
96	2356	2142	1977	1842	1627	1978	1908	1643	1570	1565
97	2374	2157	1989	1854	1636	1992	1923	1651	1579	1575
98	2392	2172	2000	1866	1644	2005	1937	1659	1589	1584
99	2409	2187	2012	1878	1653	2019	1952	1668	1598	1594

Data are kcal/24 hours.

The deviation from the predicted value may be greater at the extremes of body composition. There are limited data on the BMR of individuals with body weights greater than 80 kg.

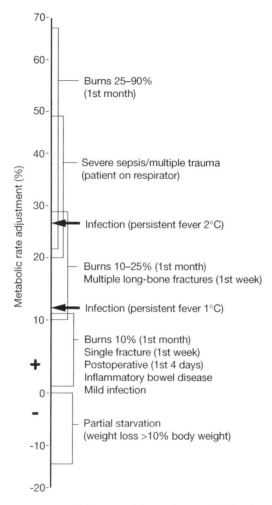

Figure 4 Elia nomogram, providing a guide to the required adjustment in BMR for the level of metabolic stress. From Elia (1990). Reproduced with permission.

Stress factors

A nomogram (Figure 4) and a table of stress factors showing stress factors over a range of certain conditions (Table 5.3) are presented. It is best to use the lower end of the range and monitor and adjust as necessary. Stress factors should be used with caution due to the risk of overfeeding, especially in the acute phase.

Table 5.3 Stress factors for some clinical conditions. Todorovic and Micklewright (2004). Reproduced with permission.

Condition	Stress factor (% BMR)
Brain injury:	
Acute (ventilated and sedated)	0–30
Recovery	5–50
Cerebral haemorrhage	30
CVA	5
COPD	15–20
Infection	25–45
IBD	0–10
Intensive care:	
Ventilated	0–10
Septic	20–60
Leukaemia	25–34
Lymphoma	0–25
Pancreatitis:	
Chronic	3
Acute	10
Sepsis/abscess	20
Solid tumours	0–20
Transplantation	20
Surgery:	
Uncomplicated	5–20
Complicated	25–40

Factors for activity and dietary-induced thermogenesis

Table 5.4 Combined factors for activity and dietary-induced thermogenesis.

Bed-bound, immobile	+10%
Bed-bound, mobile or sitting	+15–20%
Mobile, on ward	+25%

References

Department of Health (DH). *Dietary Reference Values for Food Energy and Nutrients for the UK.* Report of the Panel on Dietary Reference Values of the Committee on Medical Aspects of Food Policy. Report on Health and Social Subjects 41. London: HMSO, 1991.

Elia M. Artificial nutritional support. *Medicine International* 1990; **82**: 3392–3396.

Todorovic VE, Micklewright A (eds). *A Pocket Guide to Clinical Nutrition*, 3rd edn. Parenteral and Enteral Nutrition Group (PENG) of the British Dietetic Association. PEN Group Publications, 2004 (for availability see www.peng.org.uk).

Appendix 6 Clinical chemistry

Millimoles, milligrams and milliequivalents

Millimoles

1 millimole (mmol) = atomic weight in mg

To convert:
mg to mmol   Divide mg by the atomic weight
mmol to mg   Multiply mmol by the atomic weight

Milliequivalents

1 milliequivalent (mEq) = atomic weight in mg divided by the valency

To convert:
mg to mEq   (mg × valency)/atomic weight
mEq to mg   (mEq × atomic weight)/valency

For minerals with a valency of 1, mEq = mmol
For minerals with a valency of 2, mEq = mmol × 2

Osmolarity and osmolality

Osmolality is the number of osmotically active particles (milliosmoles) in a *kilogram* of *solvent*. Osmolarity is the number of osmotically active particles in a *litre* of *solution* (i.e. solvent + solute).

In body fluids, there is only a small difference between the two. However, in commercially prepared feeds, osmolality is always much higher than osmolarity. Osmolality is therefore the preferred term for comparing the potential hypertonic effect of liquid diets (although, in practice, it is often osmolarity which is stated).

The osmolality of a liquid feed is considerably influenced by the content of amino acids and electrolytes such as sodium and potassium. Carbohydrates with a small particle size (e.g. simple sugars) increase osmolality more than complex carbohydrates with a higher molecular weight. Fats do not increase the osmolality of solutions because of their insolubility in water.

The osmolality of plasma is normally in the range 280–300 mosmol/kg and the body attempts to keep the osmolality of the contents of the stomach and intestine at an isotonic level. It does this by producing intestinal secretions which dilute a concentrated meal or drink. If enteral feeds with a high osmolality are administered, large quantities of intestinal secretions will be produced rapidly in order to reduce the osmolality. In order to avoid diarrhoea, it is therefore important to administer such feeds slowly; the number of mosmoles given per unit of time is more important than the number of mosmoles per unit of volume.

Appendices

Table 6.1 Atomic weights and valencies of some minerals and trace elements.

Mineral	Atomic weight	Valency
Sodium	23.0	1
Potassium	39.0	1
Phosphorus	31.0	2
Calcium	40.0	2
Magnesium	24.3	2
Chlorine	35.4	1
Sulphur	32.0	2
Zinc	65.4	2

Table 6.2 Mineral content of compounds and solutions.

Solution/compound	Mineral content	
1 g sodium chloride	393 mg Na	(17.1 mmol Na$^+$)
1 g sodium bicarbonate	274 mg Na	(12 mmol Na$^+$)
1 g potassium bicarbonate	390 mg K	(10 mmol K$^+$)
1 g calcium chloride (dihydrate)	273 mg Ca	(6.8 mmol Ca^{2+})
1 g calcium carbonate	400 mg Ca	(10 mmol Ca^{2+})
1 g calcium gluconate	89 mg Ca	(2.2 mmol Ca^{2+})
1 litre normal saline	3450 mg Na	(150 mmol Na$^+$)

Table 6.3 Conversion factors for millimoles, milligrams and milliequivalents.

Mineral	mg/mmol		mg/mEq		mmol/mEq	
	mg =	mmol =	mg =	mEq =	mmol =	mEq =
Sodium	mmol × 23	mg ÷ 23	mEq × 23	mg ÷ 23	mEq	mmol
Potassium	mmol × 39	mg ÷ 39	mEq × 39	mg ÷ 39	mEq	mmol
Phosphorus	mmol × 31	mg ÷ 31	mEq × 15.5	mg ÷ 15.5	mEq ÷ 2	mmol × 2
Calcium	mmol × 40	mg ÷ 40	mEq × 20	mg ÷ 20	mEq ÷ 2	mmol × 2
Magnesium	mmol × 24.3	mg ÷ 24.3	mEq × 12.15	mg ÷ 12.15	mEq ÷ 2	mmol × 2
Chlorine	mmol × 35.4	mg ÷ 35.4	mEq × 35.4	mg ÷ 35.4	mEq	mmol
Sulphur	mmol × 32	mg ÷ 32	mEq × 16	mg ÷ 16	mEq ÷ 2	mmol × 2
Zinc	mmol × 65.4	mg ÷ 65.4	mEq × 32.7	mg ÷ 32.7	mEq ÷ 2	mmol × 2

Biochemical and haematological reference ranges

The results of laboratory tests are interpreted by comparison with reference or normal ranges. These are usually defined as the mean ± 2 SD (standard deviation), which assumes a Gaussian or normal (symmetrical) type distribution (Figure 5). Unfortunately, most biological data have a skewed rather than a symmetrical distribution and more complex statistical calculations are required to define the reference ranges.

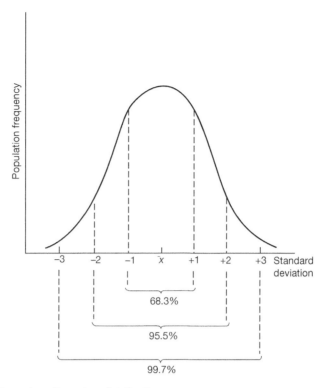

Figure 5 Normal or Gaussian distribution curve.

The reference ranges as defined usually include approximately 95% of the normal 'healthy' population; consequently, 5% of this population will have values outside the reference range but cannot be said to be abnormal. The use of reference ranges may be illustrated by taking the reference range of blood urea as 3.3–6.7 mmol/l. Approximately 95% of the normal 'healthy' population would come within these limits. However, it would be wrong to interpret a value of 6.4 mmol/l as normal while assuming a value of 7.0 mmol/l to be abnormal. Nature 'abhors abrupt transitions', so there is no clear-cut division between 'normal' and 'abnormal'. This applies equally well to body weight and height and also to measurements undertaken in the laboratory.

The majority of the normal 'healthy' population will have results close to the mean value for the population as a whole and all values will be distributed around that mean. Therefore, the probability that a value is abnormal increases the further it is from the mean value (Figure 6).

A variety of factors can cause variation in the biochemical and haematological constituents present within the blood. These can be conveniently divided into factors causing variation within an individual and those causing variation between groups of individuals.

Appendices

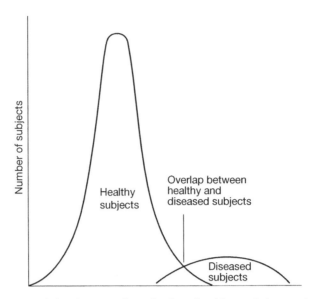

Figure 6 Theoretical distribution of results from healthy and diseased subjects.

Variations within individuals

The following factors can cause significant variation in clinical biochemical and haematological data and should be considered when interpreting individual results.

Diet
Variation in diet can affect the levels of triglycerides, cholesterol, glucose, urea and other blood constituents.

Drugs
These can have significant effects on a number of biochemical determinations, often resulting from secondary effects on sensitive organs, e.g. liver, kidney and endocrine glands. Steroids, including oral contraceptives, can cause variations in a number of biochemical and haematological parameters, including a reduction in albumin, increases in several carrier proteins, e.g. transcortin, thyroxine-binding globulin, caeruloplasmin and transferrin, and also increases in coagulation factors, e.g. fibrinogen, factor VII and factor X.

Menstrual cycle
Several biochemical constituents show marked variations with the phase of the cycle; these include the pituitary gonadotrophins, ovarian steroids and their metabolites. There is also a marked fall in plasma iron just before and during menstruation. This is probably caused by hormonal changes rather than blood loss.

Muscular exercise
Moderate exercise can cause increases in levels of potassium, together with a number of enzymes including aspartate transferase, lactate dehydrogenase, creatine kinase and hydroxybutyrate dehydrogenase.

Posture
Significant differences in the concentration of many blood constituents may be obtained by collecting blood samples from ambulant compared with recumbent individuals.

The red cell and white cell counts, together with the concentration of proteins (e.g. albumin, immunoglobulins) and protein-bound substances (e.g. calcium, cholesterol, T_4, cortisol), may decrease by up to 15% following 30 minutes of recumbency. This is probably due to fluid redistribution within the body. Hospitalised patients usually have their blood samples collected early in the morning following overnight recumbency, and consequently have significantly lower values than the normal ambulant (outpatient) population.

Stress
Both emotional and physical stress can alter circulating biochemical constituents, causing increases in the levels of pituitary hormones [e.g. adrenocorticotropic hormone (ACTH), prolactin, growth hormone] and adrenal steroids (cortisol).

Time of day
Some substances exhibit a marked circadian (diurnal) variation which is independent of meals or other activities, e.g. serum cortisol, iron and the amino acids tyrosine, phenylalanine and tryptophan. Cortisol levels are at their highest in the morning (9 am) and at their lowest levels at midnight, while iron concentration may decrease by 50% between the morning and evening. Plasma phenylalanine levels are at their lowest after midnight and reach their highest concentrations between 8.30 and 10.30 am.

Variations between groups of individuals

Several factors influence the reference values quoted for individuals. These include age, sex and race.

Age
The blood levels of many biochemical and haematological constituents are age related; these include haemoglobin, total leucocyte count, creatinine, urea, inorganic phosphate and many enzymes, e.g. alkaline phosphatase, creatine kinase and γ-glutamyl transferase. Haemoglobin levels and total leucocyte counts are highest in the newborn and gradually decrease through childhood, reaching the adult reference range at puberty. As creatinine is related to muscle mass, paediatric reference ranges are lower than those of adults. Urea levels rise slightly with age but this may well indicate impaired renal function. Alkaline phosphatase activity and inorganic phosphate levels are at their highest during childhood, reaching peak levels at puberty.

Gender

Many biochemical and haematological parameters show concentration differences which are sex dependent, including creatinine, iron, urea and the various sex hormones. Ferritin, haemoglobin and red cell counts are slightly higher in males than in females. Creatinine and urea levels are 15–20% lower in premenopausal females than in males. Premenopausal females also have lower serum iron levels than males, but after the menopause iron levels are similar in both sexes.

Race

Racial differences have been reported in some biochemical constituents, including cholesterol and protein. The reference ranges for cholesterol are higher in Europeans than in similar groups of Japanese. Similarly, the Bantu Africans have higher serum globulins than corresponding Europeans. African and Middle-Eastern individuals have lower total leucocyte and neutrophil counts than other races. Some of these racial differences are probably genetic in origin, although the environment and diet may also be contributory factors.

Laboratory variations

Methods of analysis and standardisations vary considerably from laboratory to laboratory. These differences will influence the quoted reference ranges, and therefore readers are advised to use only those quoted by their local laboratory. Local reference ranges may be at variance with the levels quoted in the following tables.

Correction of serum calcium for low albumin

Corrected serum calcium level (mmol/l)

$$= \text{measured serum calcium (mmol/l)} + \left(\frac{40 - \text{measured albumin}}{40} \right)$$

An alternative (and possibly more accurate) equation is:

Corrected serum calcium level (mmol/l)

$$= \text{measured serum calcium (mmol/l)} + \left[\left(40 - \text{measured albumin} \right) \times 0.02 \right]$$

To be even more accurate, the serum protein level should also be considered:

Corrected serum calcium level (mmol/l)

$$= \text{measured serum calcium (mmol/l)} + \left[\left(72 - \text{measured protein} \right) \times 0.02 \right]$$

This corrected calcium value should be added to that obtained from the correction for low albumin, and a mean of the two levels obtained, calculated to two decimal places.

Table 6.4 Serum/plasma levels: general biochemistry.

Blood constituent	Gender	Range	Units
Albumin		35–45	g/l
Bicarbonate		22–32	mmol/l
Bilirubin		<17	μmol/l
Calcium		2.25–2.65	mmol/l
Chloride		95–105	mmol/l
Creatinine		40–130	μmol/l
Glucose (fasting)		3.0–5.0	mmol/l
Inorganic phosphate		0.8–1.4	mmol/l
Magnesium		0.7–1.0	mmol/l
Osmolality		278–305	mosmol/kg
Potassium		3.5–5.0	mmol/l
Sodium		135–150	mmol/l
Total protein		60–80	g/l
Urate			
	Male	0.25–0.45	mmol/l
	Female	0.15–0.35	mmol/l
Urea		3.3–6.7	mmol/l

Table 6.5 Urine constituents.

Constituent	Range	Units
Calcium	<7.5	mmol/24 hours
Creatinine	9–18	mmol/24 hours
Inorganic phosphate	15–50	mmol/24 hours
Osmolality	50–1500	mosmol/24 hours
Potassium	40–120	mmol/24 hours
Protein	<0.50	g/24 hours
Sodium	100–250	mmol/24 hours
Urate	<3.0	mmol/24 hours
Urea	250–600	mmol/24 hours

Table 6.6 Faeces constituents.

Constituent	Range	Units
Faecal fat	<18	mmol/24 hours
Nitrogen	70–140	mmol/24 hours

Appendices

Table 6.7 Red cells.

Parameter	Age/sex	Range	Units
Haemoglobin	Male	13.5–17.5	g/dl
	Female	11.5–15.5	g/dl
	Newborn	15–21	g/dl
	3 months	9.5–12.5	g/dl
Haematocrit (packed cell Female volume; PCV)	Male	40–52	%
	Female	36–48	%
Red cell count	Male	4.5–6.3	10^{12}
	Female	4.2–5.4	10^{12}
Mean cell haemoglobin (MCH)		27–32	pg
Mean cell volume (MCV)		80–95	fl
Mean cell haemoglobin concentration (MCHC)		32–36	g/dl

Appendix 7 Abbreviations

AA	Amino acid	BDA	British Dietetic Association
AA	Arachidonic acid	BEE	Basal energy expenditure
AAA	Aromatic amino acids	BHF	British Heart Foundation
ABW	Actual body weight	BIA	Bioelectrical impedance analysis
ACE	Angiotensin-converting enzyme	BM	Bowel movement
ADH	Antidiuretic hormone	BMD	Bone mineral density
ADHD	Attention deficit hyperactivity disorder	BME	Black and minority ethnic
		BMI	Body mass index
ADI	Acceptable daily intake	BMR	Basal metabolic rate
ADL	Activities of daily living	BNF	British National Formulary
AIDS	Acquired immune deficiency syndrome	BoGH	Balance of Good Health
		BP	Blood pressure
ALA	α-Linolenic acid	BSA	Body surface area
ALP	Alkaline phospharase	BSG	British Society of Gastroenterology
ALT	Alanine aminotransferase		
ANS	Artificial nutrition support	BUN	Blood urea nitrogen
APD	Automated peritoneal dialysis	BV	Biological value
		BW	Body weight
ARDS	Acute respiratory distress syndrome	Bx	Biopsy
		Ca	Carcinoma
ARF	Acute renal failure	CABG	Coronary artery bypass graft
AST	Aspartare aminotransferase		
BAPEN	British Association for Parenteral and Enteral Nutrition	CAPD	Continuous ambulatory peritoneal dialysis
		CAT	Computed axial tomography
BCAA	Branched-chain amino acids	CATs	Complementary and alternative therapies
b.d.	Twice a day		

Appendices

CBT	Cognitive behavioural therapy	DVT	Deep vein thrombosis
CCF	Congestive cardiac failure	DXA	Dual-energy X-ray absorptiometry
CCK	Cholecystokinin	EAR	Estimated average requirement
CF	Cystic fibrosis		
CFS	Chronic fatigue syndrome	ECG	Electrocardiogram
CHD	Coronary heart disease	ECT	Electroconvulsive therapy
CHF	Congestive/chronic heart failure	EDD	Expected date of delivery
		EEE	Estimated energy expenditure
CLD	Chronic lung disease		
cm	Centimetre(s)	EEG	Electroencephalogram
CNS	Central nervous system	EER	Estimated energy requirement
CO	Cardiac output		
COAD	Chronic obstructive airways disease	EFA	Essential fatty acid
		EMA	Endomysial antibodies
COMA	Committee on Medical Aspects of Food Policy	EMG	Electromyography
		EN	Enteral nutrition
COPD	Chronic obstructive pulmonary disease	EPA	Eicosapentaenoic acid
		EPO	Erythropoietin
CP	Chronic pancreatitis	EPO	Evening primrose oil
CPD	Continuing professional development	ERAS	Enhanced recovery after surgery
CRF	Chronic renal failure	ESPEN	European Society of Enteral and Parenteral Nutrition
CRP	C-reactive protein (acute-phase protein)		
		ESR	Erythrocyte sedimentation rate
CSF	Cerebrospinal fluid		
CT	Computed tomography	ESRF	End-stage renal failure
CVA	Cardiovascular accident (stroke)	FAD	Flavin adenine dinucleotide
		FBC	Full blood count
CVD	Cardiovascular disease	FFM	Fat-free mass
CVP	Central venous pressure	FFQ	Food frequency questionnaire
CVS	Cardiovascular system		
DAFNE	Dose Adjustment for Normal Eating	FH	Familial hypercholesterolaemia
DCCT	Diabetes Control and Complications Trial	FH	Family history
		FHF	Fulminant hepatic failure
DD	Diverticular disease	FHS	Food hypersensitivity
DEXA	Dual-energy X-ray absorptiometry	FTD	Frontal temporal dementia
		FTT	Failure to thrive
DH	Dermatitis herpetiformis	FVC	Forced vital capacity
DIT	Dietary induced thermogenesis	g	Gram(s)
		GDA	Guideline daily amounts
DM	Diabetes mellitus	GE	Gross energy
DMUK	Diabetes UK	GF	Gluten-free
DNA	Did not attend	GFR	Glomerular filtration rate
DRI	Dietary reference intake	GGT	Gamma glutamyl transferase
DRV	Dietary reference value	GI	Gastrointestinal
D + V	Diarrhoea and vomiting	GI	Glycaemic index

GL	Glucose load	K/DOQI	Kidney Disease Outcomes Quality Initiative
GLA	γ-Linolenic acid		
GM	Genetically modified	kg	Kilogram(s)
GP	General practitioner	kJ	Kilojoule(s)
GRV	Gastric residual volume	l	Litre(s)
GTT	Glucose tolerance test	LBM	Lean body mass
HAART	Highly active anti-retroviral therapy	LBV	Low biological value
		LBW	Low birth weight
Hb	Haemoglobin	LCP	Long-chain polyunsaturated fatty acid
HbA$_{1C}$	Glycosylated haemoglobin A$_{1C}$		
		LCT	Long-chain triglyceride
HBV	Hepatitis B	LDL	Low-density lipoprotein
HBV	High biological value	LFT	Liver function tests
HCV	Hepatitis C	LRNI	Lower reference nutrient intake
HD	Huntingdon's disease		
HDL	High-density lipoprotein	m	Metre(s)
HDU	High dependency unit	MAC	Mid-arm circumference
hGH	Recombinant growth hormone	MAMC	Mid-arm muscle circumference
HIV	Human immunodeficiency virus	MAOI	Monoamine oxidase inhibitor
		MCT	Medium-chain triglyceride
HLA	Human leucocyte antigen	MCV	Mean corpuscular volume
HPC	Health Professions Council	MDT	Multi-disciplinary team
HPN	Home parenteral nutrition	ME	Metabolisable energy
HRT	Hormone replacement therapy	ME	Myalgic encephalomyopathy
		mEq	Milliequivalent(s)
IBD	Inflammatory bowel disease	mg	Milligram(s)
IBS	Irritable bowel syndrome	MG	Myasthenia gravis
IBW	Ideal body weight	MI	Meconium ileus
ICP	Integrated care pathway	MI	Motivational interviewing
ICP	Intracranial pressure	MI	Myocardial infarction
ICU	Intensive care unit	MIMS	Monthly Index of Medical Specialities
IDDM	Insulin-dependent diabetes mellitus (now called type 1 diabetes)		
		MJ	Megajoule(s)
		ml	Millilitre(s)
IDPN	Intra-dialytic parenteral nutrition	mmHg	Millimetres of mercury
		mmol	Millimole(s)
IGT	Impaired glucose tolerance	MNA	Mini-nutritional assessment
i.m.	Intramuscular	MND	Motor neurone disease
I/O	Intake and output	MNDA	Motor Neurone Disease Association
i.p.	Intraperitoneal		
ITU	Intensive therapy unit	MODY	Maturity onset diabetes of the young
IU/i.u.	International units		
IUGR	Intrauterine growth restricted	MOF	Multiple organ failure
i.v.	Intravascular/intravenous	mosmol	Milliosmole(s)
IVIG	Intravenous immunoglobulin	MRI	Magnetic resonance imaging
kcal	Kilocalorie(s)	MS	Mitral stenosis

MS	Multiple sclerosis	PBC	Primary biliary cirrhosis
MSG	Monosodium glutamate	PBM	Peak bone mass
MSU	Midstream urine	PCOS	Polycystic ovary syndrome
MUAC	Mid-upper arm circumference	PCP	*Pneumocystis carinii* pneumonia
MUFA	Monounsaturated fatty acid	PCT	Primary Care Trust
MUST	Malnutrition Universal Screening Tool	PCV	Packed cell volume
		PD	Parkinson's disease
N	Nitrogen	PD	Peritoneal dialysis
n-3	Omega-3 (fatty acids)	PDUO	Previous day's urinary output
n-6	Omega-6 (fatty acids)	PE	Physical examination
NAD	Nothing abnormal detected	PE	Plasma exchange
NAGE	Nutrition Advisory Group for Elderly People	PE	Pulmonary embolism
		PEG	Percutaneous endoscopic gastrostomy
NAO	National Association of Obesity	PEJ	Percutaneous endoscopic jejeunostomy
NAS	No added salt	PEM	Protein-energy malnutrition
NBM	Nil-by-mouth	PENG	Parenteral and Enteral Nutrition Group (of the British Dietetic Association)
NDNS	National Diet and Nutrition Survey		
NFS	National Food Survey	PERT	Pancreatic enzyme replacement therapy
NG	Nasogastric		
NHS	National Health Service	PET	Pre-eclampsia toxaemia
NHS-QIS	NHS Quality Improvement Scotland	PF	Peak flow
		PI	Pancreatic insufficient
NICE	National Institute for Health and Clinical Excellence	PMA	Progressive muscular atrophy
		PMH	Past medical history
NIDDM	Non-insulin dependent diabetes mellitus (now called type 2 diabetes)	PMS	Premenstrual syndrome
		PN	Parenteral nutrition (or total parenteral nutrition – TPN)
NMR	Nuclear magnetic resonance		
NRI	Nutrition risk index	p.o.	Per os (by mouth)
NRV	Nutrient reference value	PPF	Plasma protein fraction
NSAID	Non-steroidal anti-inflammatory drug	PPH	Post-partum haemorrhage
		PRA	Prealbumin (acute-phase protein)
NSF	National Service Framework		
NSP	Non-starch polysaccharide	PRG	Percutaneous radiological gastrostomy
N + V	Nausea and vomiting		
OA	Osteoarthritis	PRI	Population reference intake
OA	On admission	prn	When required
o.d.	Every day/once a day	PSE	Portal systemic encephalopathy
OE	On examination		
OGTT	Oral glucose tolerance test	PTH	Parathyroid hormone
OHA	Oral hypoglycaemic agent	PU	Peptic ulcer
OT	Occupational therapist	PUFA	Polyunsaturated fatty acid
PAL	Physical activity level	PUO	Pyrexia of unknown origin
PAR	Physical activity ratio	PVD	Peripheral vascular disease

Appendices

PVS	Persistent vegetative state		SLE	Systemic lupus erythematosus
QAA	Quality Assurance Agency		SLT	Speech and language therapist
q.d.	Every day			
q.d.s.	Four times a day		SMART	Specific, Measurable, Achievable, Relevant and Time specific
q.h.	Every hour			
QUID	Quantitative ingredients declaration			
RA	Rheumatoid arthritis		SOA	Swelling of ankles
RAST	Radioallergosorbant test		SOB	Shortness of breath
RBC	Red blood cell/count		T^4	Thyroxine
RBP	Retinol-binding protein		TB	Tuberculosis
RBS	Random blood sugar		TBI	Traumatic brain injury
RCP	Royal College of Physicians		TBP	Total body protein
RCT	Randomised controlled trial		TBW	Total body water
RD	Registered dietitian		TDS	Total diet survey
RDA	Recommended daily amount/ recommended dietary allowance		t.d.s.	Three times a day
			TEE	Total energy expenditure
			TIA	Transient ischaemic attack
RDI	Reference/recommended daily intake		TIBC	Total iron-binding capacity
			TNF	Tumour necrosis factor
RE	Retinol equivalents		TPN	Total parenteral nutrition (now called PN)
REE	Resting energy expenditure			
RFT	Respiratory function tests		TSF	Triceps skinfold thickness
RMR	Resting metabolic rate		TSH	Thyroid stimulating hormone
RNI	Reference nutrient intake		Tx	Treatment/therapy
RQ	Respiratory quotient		TUFA	Trans unsaturated fatty acid
RR	Relative risk		UA	Urinalysis
RRT	Renal replacement therapy		UC	Ulcerative colitis
RS	Resistant starch		U + E	Urea and electrolytes
RTA	Renal tubular acidosis		UKM	Urea kinetic modelling
RTA	Road traffic accident		UKPDS	United Kingdom Prospective Diabetes Study Group
RTF	Ready-to-feed			
RUQ	Right upper quadrant		UL	Tolerable upper limit
R_x	Recommended therapy		UO	Urinary output
SBS	Short bowel syndrome		UTI	Urinary tract infection
SCFA	Short-chain fatty acid		VLBW	Very low birth weight
SCI	Spinal cord injury		VLCD	Very low calorie diet
s.d.	Standard deviation		VLDL	Very low-density lipoprotein
SFA	Saturated fatty acid		WCC	White cell count
SGA	Small for gestational age		WHO	World Health Organization
SGA	Subjective global assessment		μg	Microgram(s)
SGI	Subjective global index		5-HT	5-Hydroxytryptamine (serotonin)
SI	Small intestine			
SIGN	Scottish Intercollegiate Guidelines Network		#	Fracture

The appendices: tools

Appendix 8 Algorithm for treating malnutrition: decision-making tool

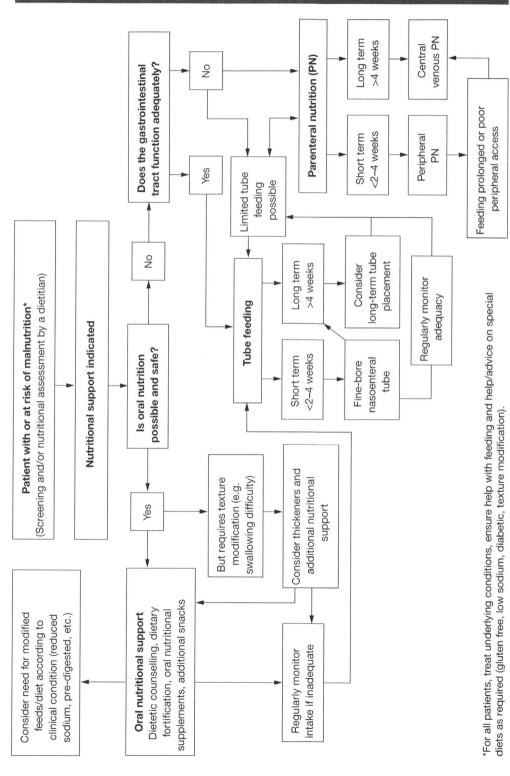

*For all patients, treat underlying conditions, ensure help with feeding and help/advice on special diets as required (gluten free, low sodium, diabetic, texture modification).

Appendix 9 Malnutrition universal screening tool ('MUST')

Reproduced with kind permission of BAPEN from *The 'MUST' Report. Nutritional Screening of Adults: A Multidisciplinary Responsibility. Development and Use of the Malnutrition Universal Screening Tool (MUST) for Adults.* Editor: Professor Marinos Elia. BAPEN, 2003. ISBN 1-899467-70-X.

'MUST'

'MUST' is a five-step screening tool to identify **adults**, who are malnourished, at risk of malnutrition (undernutrition), or obese. It also includes management guidelines which can be used to develop a care plan. It is for use in hospitals, community and other care settings and can be used by all care workers.

This guide contains:

- A flow chart showing the 5 steps to use for screening and management
- BMI chart
- Weight loss tables
- Alternative measurements when BMI cannot be obtained by measuring weight and height

The 5 'MUST' steps

Step 1: measure height and weight to get a BMI score using chart provided. *If unable to obtain height and weight, use the alternative procedures shown in this guide.*

Step 2: note percentage unplanned weight loss and score using tables provided.

Step 3: establish acute disease effect and score.

Step 4: add scores from steps 1, 2 and 3 together to obtain overall risk of malnutrition.

Step 5: use management guidelines and/or local policy to develop care plan.

Please refer to *The 'MUST' Explanatory Booklet* for more information when weight and height cannot be measured, and when screening patient groups in which extra care in interpretation is needed (e.g. those with fluid disturbances, plaster casts, amputations, critical illness and pregnant or lactating women). The booklet can also be used for training. See *The 'MUST' Report* for supporting evidence. Please note that 'MUST' has not been designed to detect deficiencies or excessive intakes of vitamins and minerals and is of **use only in adults**.

Appendices

Step 1: BMI score (and BMI)

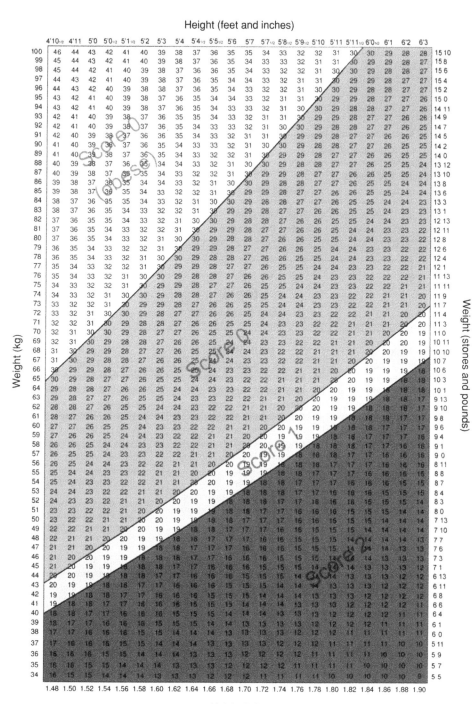

Height (feet and inches)

Weight (kg)

Weight (stones and pounds)

Height (m)

Appendices

Note: The black lines denote the exact cut off points (30, 20 and 18.5 kg/m^2), figures on the chart have been rounded to the nearest whole number.

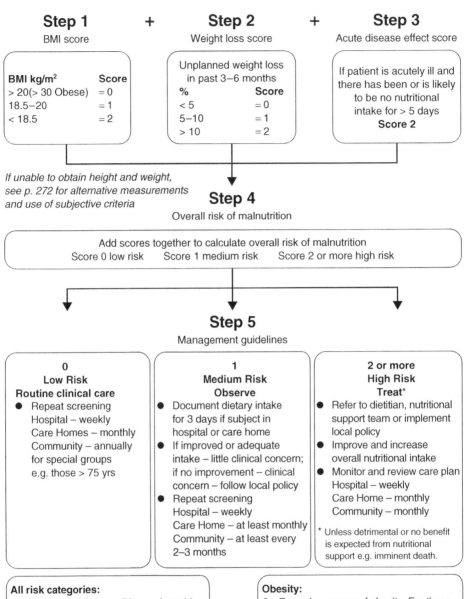

Step 1
+
Step 2
+
Step 3

BMI score

Weight loss score

Acute disease effect score

BMI kg/m²	Score
> 20(> 30 Obese)	= 0
18.5–20	= 1
< 18.5	= 2

Unplanned weight loss
in past 3–6 months

%	Score
< 5	= 0
5–10	= 1
> 10	= 2

If patient is acutely ill and
there has been or is likely
to be no nutritional
intake for > 5 days
Score 2

*If unable to obtain height and weight,
see p. 272 for alternative measurements
and use of subjective criteria*

Step 4
Overall risk of malnutrition

Add scores together to calculate overall risk of malnutrition
Score 0 low risk   Score 1 medium risk   Score 2 or more high risk

Step 5
Management guidelines

0	1	2 or more
Low Risk	**Medium Risk**	**High Risk**
Routine clinical care	**Observe**	**Treat***
● Repeat screening Hospital – weekly Care Homes – monthly Community – annually for special groups e.g. those > 75 yrs	● Document dietary intake for 3 days if subject in hospital or care home ● If improved or adequate intake – little clinical concern; if no improvement – clinical concern – follow local policy ● Repeat screening Hospital – weekly Care Home – at least monthly Community – at least every 2–3 months	● Refer to dietitian, nutritional support team or implement local policy ● Improve and increase overall nutritional intake ● Monitor and review care plan Hospital – weekly Care Home – monthly Community – monthly * Unless detrimental or no benefit is expected from nutritional support e.g. imminent death.

All risk categories:
● Treat underlying condition and provide help and advice on food choices, eating and drinking when necessary.
● Record malnutrition risk category.
● Record need for special diets and follow local policy.

Obesity:
● Record presence of obesity. For those with underlying conditions, these are generally controlled before the treatment of obesity.

Re-assess subjects identified at risk as they move through care settings

See The 'MUST' Explanatory Booklet for further details and The 'MUST' Report for supporting evidence

Step 2: weight loss score

Weight before weight loss (st lb)

Weight	Score 0 Wt Loss <5%	Score 1 Wt Loss 5–10%	Score 2 Wt Loss >10%
34 kg	<1.70	1.70–3.40	>3.40
36 kg	<1.80	1.80–3.60	>3.60
38 kg	<1.90	1.90–3.80	>3.80
40 kg	<2.00	2.00–4.00	>4.00
42 kg	<2.10	2.10–4.20	>4.20
44 kg	<2.20	2.20–4.40	>4.40
46 kg	<2.30	2.30–4.60	>4.60
48 kg	<2.40	2.40–4.80	>4.80
50 kg	<2.50	2.50–5.00	>5.00
52 kg	<2.60	2.60–5.20	>5.20
54 kg	<2.70	2.70–5.40	>5.40
56 kg	<2.80	2.80–5.60	>5.60
58 kg	<2.90	2.90–5.80	>5.80
60 kg	<3.00	3.00–6.00	>6.00
62 kg	<3.10	3.10–6.20	>6.20
64 kg	<3.20	3.20–6.40	>6.40
66 kg	<3.30	3.30–6.60	>6.60
68 kg	<3.40	3.40–6.80	>6.80
70 kg	<3.50	3.50–7.00	>7.00
72 kg	<3.60	3.60–7.20	>7.20
74 kg	<3.70	3.70–7.40	>7.40
76 kg	<3.80	3.80–7.60	>7.60
78 kg	<3.90	3.90–7.80	>7.80
80 kg	<4.00	4.00–8.00	>8.00
82 kg	<4.10	4.10–8.20	>8.20
84 kg	<4.20	4.20–8.40	>8.40
86 kg	<4.30	4.30–8.60	>8.60
88 kg	<4.40	4.40–8.80	>8.80
90 kg	<4.50	4.50–9.00	>9.00
92 kg	<4.60	4.60–9.20	>9.20
94 kg	<4.70	4.70–9.40	>9.40
96 kg	<4.80	4.80–9.60	>9.60
98 kg	<4.90	4.90–9.80	>9.80
100 kg	<5.00	5.00–10.00	>10.00
102 kg	<5.10	5.10–10.20	>10.20
104 kg	<5.20	5.20–10.40	>10.40
106 kg	<5.30	5.30–10.60	>10.60
108 kg	<5.40	5.40–10.80	>10.80
110 kg	<5.50	5.50–11.00	>11.00
112 kg	<5.60	5.60–11.20	>11.20
114 kg	<5.70	5.70–11.40	>11.40
116 kg	<5.80	5.80–11.60	>11.60
118 kg	<5.90	5.90–11.80	>11.80
120 kg	<6.00	6.00–12.00	>12.00
122 kg	<6.10	6.10–12.20	>12.20
124 kg	<6.20	6.20–12.40	>12.40
126 kg	<6.30	6.30–12.60	>12.60

Weight before weight loss (kg)

Weight	Score 0 Wt Loss <5%	Score 1 Wt Loss 5–10%	Score 2 Wt Loss >10%
5st 4lb	<4 lb	4 lb–7 lb	>7 lb
5st 7lb	<4 lb	4 lb–8 lb	>8 lb
5st 11lb	<4 lb	4 lb–8 lb	>8 lb
6st	<4 lb	4 lb–8 lb	>8 lb
6st 4lb	<4 lb	4 lb–9 lb	>9 lb
6st 7lb	<5 lb	5 lb–9 lb	>9 lb
6st 11lb	<5 lb	5 lb–10 lb	>10 lb
7st	<5 lb	5 lb–10 lb	>10 lb
7st 4lb	<5 lb	5 lb–10 lb	>10 lb
7st 7lb	<5 lb	5 lb–11 lb	>11 lb
7st 11lb	<5 lb	5 lb–11 lb	>11 lb
8st	<6 lb	6 lb–11 lb	>11 lb
8st 4lb	<6 lb	6 lb–12 lb	>12 lb
8st 7lb	<6 lb	6 lb–12 lb	>12 lb
8st 11lb	<6 lb	6 lb–12 lb	>12 lb
9st	<6 lb	6 lb–13 lb	>13 lb
9st 4lb	<7 lb	7 lb–13 lb	>13 lb
9st 7lb	<7 lb	7 lb–13 lb	>13 lb
9st 11lb	<7 lb	7 lb–1st 0 lb	>1st 0 lb
10st	<7 lb	7 lb–1st 0 lb	>1st 0 lb
10st 4lb	<7 lb	7 lb–1st 0 lb	>1st 0 lb
10st 7lb	<7 lb	7 lb–1st 1 lb	>1st 1 lb
10st 11lb	<8 lb	8 lb–1st 1 lb	>1st 1 lb
11st	<8 lb	8 lb–1st 1 lb	>1st 1 lb
11st 4lb	<8 lb	8 lb–1st 2 lb	>1st 2 lb
11st 7lb	<8 lb	8 lb–1st 2 lb	>1st 2 lb
11st 11lb	<8 lb	8 lb–1st 3 lb	>1st 3 lb
12st	<8 lb	8 lb–1st 3 lb	>1st 3 lb
12st 4lb	<9 lb	9 lb–1st 3 lb	>1st 3 lb
12st 7lb	<9 lb	9 lb–1st 4 lb	>1st 4 lb
12st 11lb	<9 lb	9 lb–1st 4 lb	>1st 4 lb
13st	<9 lb	9 lb–1st 4 lb	>1st 4 lb
13st 4lb	<9 lb	9 lb–1st 5 lb	>1st 5 lb
13st 7lb	<9 lb	9 lb–1st 5 lb	>1st 5 lb
13st 11lb	<10 lb	10 lb–1st 5 lb	>1st 5 lb
14st	<10 lb	10 lb–1st 6 lb	>1st 6 lb
14st 4lb	<10 lb	10 lb–1st 6 lb	>1st 6 lb
14st 7lb	<10 lb	10 lb–1st 6 lb	>1st 6 lb
14st 11lb	<10 lb	10 lb–1st 7 lb	>1st 7 lb
15st	<11 lb	11 lb–1st 7 lb	>1st 7 lb
15st 4lb	<11 lb	11 lb–1st 7 lb	>1st 7 lb
15st 7lb	<11 lb	11 lb–1st 8 lb	>1st 8 lb
15st 11lb	<11 lb	11 lb–1st 8 lb	>1st 8 lb
16st	<11 lb	11 lb–1st 8 lb	>1st 8 lb
16st 4lb	<11 lb	11 lb–1st 9 lb	>1st 9 lb
16st 7lb	<12 lb	12 lb–1st 9 lb	>1st 9 lb

Appendices

Alternative measurements and considerations

Step 1: BMI (body mass index)

If height cannot be measured

- Use recently documented or self-reported height (if reliable and realistic).
- If the subject does not know or is unable to report their height, use one of the alternative measurements to estimate height (ulna, knee height or demispan).

If height and weight cannot be obtained

- Use mid-upper arm circumference (MUAC) measurement to estimate BMI category.

Step 2: Recent unplanned weight loss

If recent weight loss cannot be calculated, use self-reported weight loss (if reliable and realistic).

Subjective criteria

If height, weight or BMI cannot be obtained, the following criteria which relate to them can assist your professional judgement of the subject's nutritional risk.

(1) BMI

- Clinical impression – thin, acceptable weight, overweight. Obvious wasting (very thin) and obesity (very overweight) can also be noted.

(2) Unplanned weight loss

- Clothes and/or jewellery have become loose fitting (weight loss).
- History of decreased food intake, reduced appetite or swallowing problems over 3–6 months and underlying disease or psycho-social/physical disabilities likely to cause weight loss.

(3) Acute disease effect

- No nutritional intake or likelihood of no intake for more than 5 days.

Further details on taking alternative measurements, special circumstances and subjective criteria can be found in The 'MUST' Explanatory Booklet. A copy can be downloaded at www.bapen.org.uk or purchased from the BAPEN office. The full evidence-base for 'MUST' is contained in The 'MUST' Report which is also available from the BAPEN office:

Secure Hold Business Centre, Studley Road, Redditch, Worcs BN98 7LG. Tel: 01527 457850.

Alternative measurements: instructions and tables

If height cannot be obtained, use length of forearm (ulna) to calculate height using tables below. *(See The 'MUST' Explanatory Booklet for details of other alternative measurements (knee height and demispan) that can also be used to estimate height.)*

Estimating height from ulna length

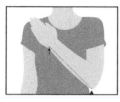

Measure between the point of the elbow (olecranon process) and the midpoint of the prominent bone of the wrist (styloid process) (left side if possible).

HEIGHT (m)	Men(< 65 years)	1.94	1.93	1.91	1.89	1.87	1.85	1.84	1.82	1.80	1.78	1.76	1.75	1.73	1.71
	Men(> 65 years)	1.87	1.86	1.84	1.82	1.81	1.79	1.78	1.76	1.75	1.73	1.71	1.70	1.68	1.67
	Ulna length (cm)	32.0	31.5	31.0	30.5	30.0	29.5	29.0	28.5	28.0	27.5	27.0	26.5	26.0	25.5
HEIGHT (m)	Women(< 65 years)	1.84	1.83	1.81	1.80	1.79	1.77	1.76	1.75	1.73	1.72	1.70	1.69	1.68	1.66
	Women(> 65 years)	1.84	1.83	1.81	1.79	1.78	1.76	1.75	1.73	1.71	1.70	1.68	1.66	1.65	1.63
HEIGHT (m)	Men(< 65 years)	1.69	1.67	1.66	1.64	1.62	1.60	1.58	1.57	1.55	1.53	1.51	1.49	1.48	1.46
	Men(> 65 years)	1.65	1.63	1.62	1.60	1.59	1.57	1.56	1.54	1.52	1.51	1.49	1.48	1.46	1.45
	Ulna length (cm)	25.0	24.5	24.0	23.5	23.0	22.5	22.0	21.5	21.0	20.5	20.0	19.5	19.0	18.5
HEIGHT (m)	Women(< 65 years)	1.65	1.63	1.62	1.61	1.59	1.58	1.56	1.55	1.54	1.52	1.51	1.50	1.48	1.47
	Women(> 65 years)	1.61	1.60	1.58	1.56	1.55	1.53	1.52	1.50	1.48	1.47	1.45	1.44	1.42	1.40

Estimating BMI category from mid-upper arm circumference (MUAC)

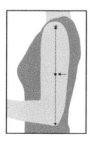

The subject's left arm should be bent at the elbow at a 90 degree angle, with the upper arm held parallel to the side of the body. Measure the distance between the bony protrusion on the shoulder (acromion) and the point of the elbow (olecranon process). Mark the midpoint.

Ask the subject to let arm hang loose and measure around the upper arm at the midpoint, making sure that the tape measure is snug but not tight.

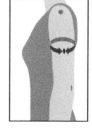

If MUAC is < 23.5 cm, BMI is likely to be   < 20 kg/m ^{2}

If MUAC is > 32.0 cm, BMI is likely to be   > 30 kg/m ^{2}

Appendix 10 Balance of good health: sensible eating tool

Fruit and vegetables
Choose a wide variety

Bread, other cereals and potatoes
Eat all types and choose high fibre kinds whenever you can

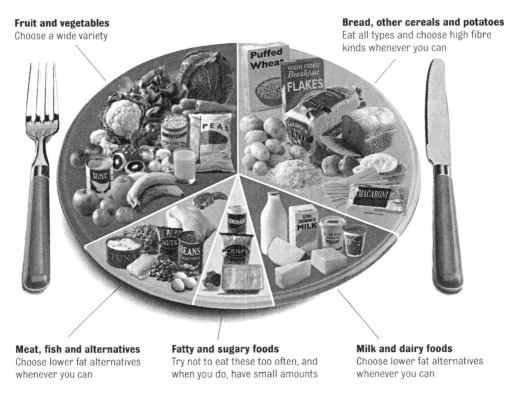

Meat, fish and alternatives
Choose lower fat alternatives whenever you can

Fatty and sugary foods
Try not to eat these too often, and when you do, have small amounts

Milk and dairy foods
Choose lower fat alternatives whenever you can

There are five main groups of valuable foods

Index

Printed and bound in the UK by
CPI Antony Rowe, Eastbourne

Printed and bound by CPI Group (UK) Ltd, Croydon, CR0 4YY

27/10/2024

14580202-0001